T0213914

Knee Arthroscopy

Olivier Courage · Simon Bertiaux
Pierre-Emmanuel Papin
Anthony Kamel

Knee Arthroscopy

How to Succeed

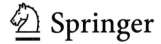 Springer

Olivier Courage
Hôpital Privé de l'Estuaire
Le Havre
France

Simon Bertiaux
Hôpital Privé de l'Estuaire
Le Havre
France

Pierre-Emmanuel Papin
Department of Orthopedics and
Traumatology
Groupe Hospitalier Intercommunal
Le Rain
Montfermeil
France

Anthony Kamel
Hôpital Privé de l'Estuaire
Le Havre
France

Original French edition published by Sauramps Medical, Montpellier, 2020
Translation from the French language edition: Comment réussir ses arthroscopies de genou? by Olivier Courage, et al., © Sauramps Medical, Montpellier, France, 2020 2020. Published by Sauramps Medical. All Rights Reserved.

ISBN 978-3-030-82832-5   ISBN 978-3-030-82830-1   (eBook)
https://doi.org/10.1007/978-3-030-82830-1

This Springer imprint is published by the registered company Springer Nature Switzerland AG
The registered company address is: Gewerbestrasse 11, 6330 Cham, Switzerland

Foreword

This book is dedicated to the sports-related surgery of the knee and describes in a very precise way the techniques recommended and used by Olivier Courage.

Dr. Courage is a very experienced surgeon who details the techniques he has been using for the last 30 years in terms of practicing surgery focused on a specific domain: ligamentous and meniscal surgery of the knee.

It is a real treatise in which the surgical technique is described step by step, allowing the reader to easily reproduce the surgical act.

The style is direct, reflecting the author's personality, and the illustrations answer the questions of surgeons who are not used to these techniques. On the other hand, experienced surgeons will find the details helpful in optimizing the progress of the procedure.

The numerous photos added to the book allow an effortless understanding of the steps of the procedure.

In addition, the objective set by the author sharing his experience and tricks with others is well achieved.

Finally, if we adopt this aphorism of Otto von Bismarck "*Fools learn from experience. I prefer to learn from the experience of others*," then we should carefully read this book and in detail that is far rewarding and original.

Caluire-et-Cuire, Lyon, France   Philippe Neyret

Preface

It has been 40 years since this art has taken off, and since then the numerous and various surgical techniques in knee arthroscopy have been well structured and explained in many reference books.

So, is this the umpteenth book that you have between your hands?

Well, NO! Here, like in the previous edition devoted to shoulder arthroscopy, the value of this book lies not in its exhaustiveness but rather in its pedagogical aspect.

It is the "Swiss knife" of the "arthroscopist" in the making, a must-have to his library.

We all started once with our loads of groping and hesitation. No one is born a master of arthroscope, even if the performance of certain actions done by an experienced physician may give, to the young generations, a false impression of their simplicity.

How can we pass these fundamentals to the vast majority of young generations in order to acquire a fine and precise surgical ability and help them avoid the errors that marked out our first knee arthroscopies?

The companionship, this active teaching approach from a master to an apprentice, of knowledge and experience gained over time, constitutes the gold standard of surgical teaching and should remain so. The objective of this collection is to get closer to this approach coming directly from one's knowledge in order to make it accessible to all, even to those who are outside the walls of the operating room.

Le Havre, France   Olivier Courage
Le Havre, France   Simon Bertiaux
Montfermeil, France   Pierre-Emmanuel Papin
Le Havre, France   Anthony Kamel

Acknowledgments

I have always been questioned about the source of my urge to teach. The answer is so simple: in 1987, I have met Bruno Locker, who, as a young resident then, helped me escape from my timidity and guided me in my arthroscopic gestures.

In conventional surgery, I have to thank Pr. Vielpeau with whom I had a perfect internship, and I feel like I have to pass to others this gift of mine.

Contrary to the first book *How to succeed a shoulder arthroscopy?* this one is a fruit of teamwork.

I am grateful to Dr. Simon Bertiaux, my colleague, who, with his new cruciate ligaments reconstruction techniques, has brought an innovative ligamentous surgery technique, allowing new dynamism and an ambulatory management to his patients. He was one of my residents, 10 years ago, and now assumes the role of a teacher. This chain of active transmission is extremely pleasant to live on a daily basis.

I also thank Pierre Emmanuel Papin, who was a resident during the writing of this book. He helped and motivated me to finish the book within the time limit with his knowledge in the photography world. He is a proof of importance of true companionship, evolution of the internship, and notably what young residents can offer to their senior teachers.

In addition, I would like to express my gratitude to all the residents who, since 2008, were formed in the "Havre Arthroscopy Surgery School" or the HASS! This association helps us reunite every year in a relaxed atmosphere to discuss newer techniques, indications, difficult cases, etc. I have to admit that this is a source of great joy for all of us and especially for me to see them evolve. The smiles on this photo tell us a lot about the reigning atmosphere!

Appreciation is also due to the operating team, the brave girls, who maintain a high technical level with that sense of humor!

Heartfelt thanks to Eden Escargooo who, thanks to his talent, adds a fun aspect to this book.

Thank you for reading the book till the end.

We invite you to visit our clinic "Hôpital Privé de l'Estuaire," where all the team awaits you.

Well, that is it folks!

Contents

1 The Basics: Patient's Positioning, Different Portals of the Knee 1
1.1 Patient Positioning 1
1.2 The Different Portals 1
1.3 The Exploration 4

**2 Meniscal Sutures: All-Inside, Out-In, and Posterior Horn
Reinsertion** 13
2.1 Overview 13
  2.1.1 The Abrasion 13
  2.1.2 The All-Inside Suture 13
  2.1.3 Out-In Technique 16

**3 The Hamstring Graft: ACL Reconstruction with Quadruple
Bundle Gracilis and Semitendinosus Tendons** 23
3.1 Overview 23
3.2 Hamstring Tendons Graft Harvesting: Anterior
  Approach 23
3.3 Femoral Tunnel: First Part 25
3.4 Tibial Tunnel 30
3.5 Femoral Tunnel: Second Part 30
3.6 Ascent, Tension Adjustment, and Transplant Fixation 31

**4 Quadruple Hamstring Graft: Single Four-Strand
Semitendinosus Tendon** 39
4.1 Overview 39
4.2 Semitendinosus Tendon Harvesting Using the
  Posterior Popliteal Fossa Approach 39
4.3 Graft Preparation 40
4.4 Femoral Tunnel, Out-In Technique 43
4.5 Tibial Tunnel 47
4.6 The Ascent, the Tension Adjustment, and Graft Fixation 48

**5 BTB Graft Technique: ACL Reconstruction Using the
Patellar Tendon** 51
5.1 Overview 51
5.2 Patellar Tendon Harvesting 51
5.3 Preparing the Femoral Intercondylar Fossa 53
5.4 Tibial Tunnel 54
5.5 Femoral Tunnel 55

5.6 Ascent, Tension Adjustment, and Transplant Fixation 56
5.7 Closure 59

6 Lateral Tenodesis: Extra-articular Reconstruction with the Fascia Lata Using a Modified Christel-Djian Technique ... 61
6.1 Overview 61
6.2 Harvesting 61
6.3 Fixation 61

7 The Posterior Cruciate Ligament: PCL Reconstruction Using the Semitendinosus 65
7.1 Overview 65
7.2 The Single Four-Strand Semitendinosus Tendon Harvesting . 65
7.3 Graft Preparation 65
7.4 A Complete Tunnel Using the Image Intensifier 65
7.5 Femoral Tunnels In-Out 67
7.6 Ascent, Tension Adjustment, and Transplant Fixation 68

8 The MPFL: Double Bundle Reconstruction Using the Gracilis with Femoral and Tibial Rigid Fixations 73
8.1 Overview 73
8.2 Patient Positioning 73
8.3 Gracilis Tendon Harvesting and Length Verification 73
8.4 Preoperative Skin Marking at the Fixation Sites 73
8.5 Patellar Tunnel Fixation with Screws 75
8.6 Femoral Fixation with a Screw in a Complete Tunnel 75

Annex A: Learning on the Simulator 79

Annex B: Graft Preparation During a Quadruple Stranded Semitendinosus Technique 83

1.1 Patient Positioning

The patient is placed in a supine position on a standard operating table, while bending the knee to 90° of ipsilateral flexion, with a knee stabilizer placed under the leg. In addition, a lateral stress post is placed beside the thigh at the tourniquet level (Figs. 1.1 and 1.2).

A variant is used for ACL reconstruction, the knee is placed in 70° of flexion rather than 90° in order to have a better exposure of the entire condylar notch, in particular the tibial footprint of the ACL.

It is always best to verify the patient's positioning before draping since changing it after will be more challenging. This is why we simulate the operation's leg positions just after the installation mainly in Cabot and knee valgus stress maneuvers (Figs. 1.3, 1.4, and 1.5). Thus, we might detect malpositioning or loosening of the braces, or we might find a table that is too low, etc.

When the exposure of the meniscus is difficult, usually the problem comes from bad positioning.

We have to think about our comfort, by avoiding standing in a twisted position in order to protect our backs.

This is why the respect of the head, hands, and screen alignment is crucial (Fig. 1.6).

In order to avoid water-soaking and a longer floor cleaning time between two interventions, we have to prevent and anticipate water flow.

This is why we place a collection bucket with the fold of the drape directed towards it. This would please the team. This is why this technique is known as "the river of love" (Fig. 1.7).

One should not forget the focus adjustment and the white balance on a compress.

The use of a tourniquet at the proximal part of the thigh is systematic except for meniscectomies.

In addition, well patient positioning is the key to success.

We can now start the intervention with serenity and explore the knee.

1.2 The Different Portals

The anterolateral portal of the scope is made in the angle formed by the lateral border of the patella, the tibial plateau, and the lateral portion of the patellar tendon, in the "soft point" and in its superior part (Fig. 1.8).

The scalpel is inclined at 45° to the horizontal aiming the intercondylar notch. The blade is oriented upwards to avoid iatrogenic lesion of the meniscus (Figs. 1.9, 1.10, and 1.11).

One trick for avoiding water loss is to make a small cut in the capsule without passing the whole blade.

The height level of the anteromedial (instrumental) portal is dictated by the principal compartment in question. For example, if we want to pass the tibial spine in order to access the

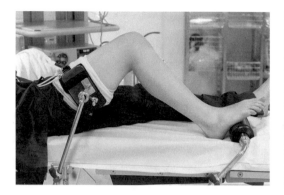

Fig. 1.1 Classic patient positioning in 90° of knee flexion

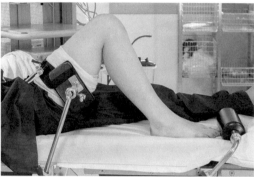

Fig. 1.2 120° of knee flexion

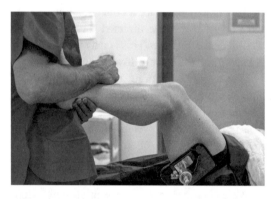

Fig. 1.3 Here in a valgus stress maneuver, the stress post is placed too low. The thigh passes over it. Hence, we should ascend the table

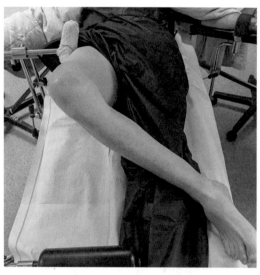

Fig. 1.4 The stress post prevents the varus positioning

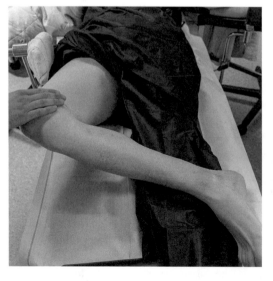

Fig. 1.5 Once the post is shifted, the varus positioning will be possible and more stress can be applied to the knee

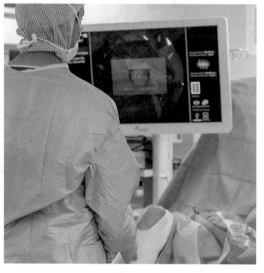

Fig. 1.6 Alignment of the head-hands-screen

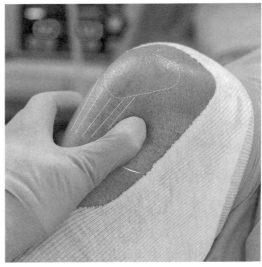

Fig. 1.8 Palpation of entry point

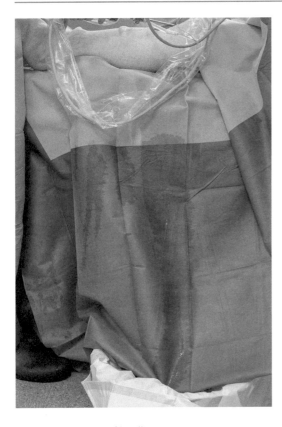

Fig. 1.7 "The river of love"

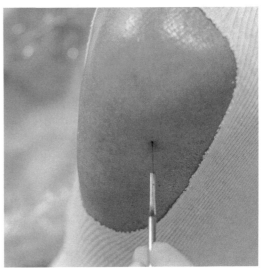

Fig. 1.10 Blade aimed at a 45° angle towards the intercondylar notch

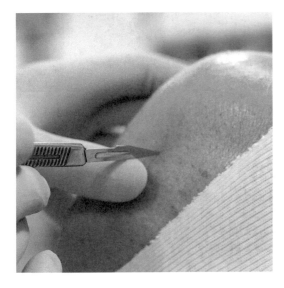

Fig. 1.9 Blade oriented upwards

posterior and middle horns of the lateral meniscus, we prefer an approach that is a little bit higher than usual and closer to the patellar tendon. Conversely, if the obstacle we want to surpass is the medial femoral condyle, we opt for a lower anteromedial portal, flush with the surface of the anterior meniscus horn.

In order to precisely locate the incision level, we can use a needle especially at the beginning of

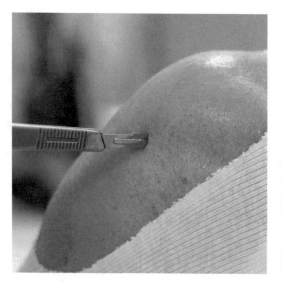

Fig. 1.11 Not forcing the entry of the blade

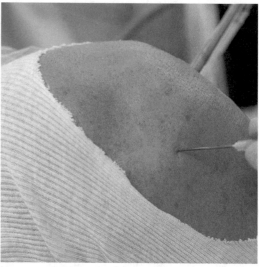

Fig. 1.12 Transillumination permits, along with palpation, to relocate the joint line level

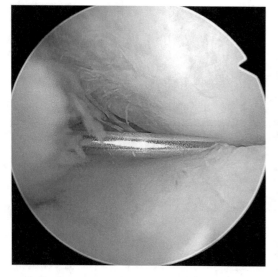

Fig. 1.13 The needle simulates the incision level

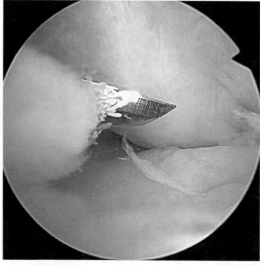

Fig. 1.14 The blade should be partially visualized

our career. The blade will be oriented towards the condyle (Figs. 1.12, 1.13, and 1.14).

If we intend to work on the two compartments, we can begin by exploring the knee in order to evaluate which compartment needs to be worked at the most, so we can adapt our anteromedial portal accordingly.

1.3   The Exploration

First, we insert the soft trocar by the anterolateral portal in a 45° horizontal inclination (in the same direction of the blade) directed towards the intercondylar notch.

Once it is blocked by the medial femoral condyle, we open the water flow to gain space, so we can introduce the trocar under the patella. We extend the knee progressively while passing the trocar under the quadricipital tendon.

The soft trocar is then removed, and the scope is introduced and locked.

The exploration has begun. We have to use the maximal visual capacities of the 30° scope. We also have to visualize systematically and successively:

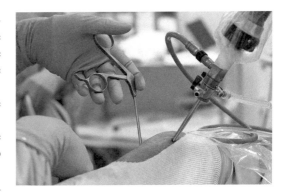

Fig. 1.15 The fingers are out of the forceps eyelets

In extension	1. Suprapatellar pouch 2. The patella 3. Intercondylar ramps 4. The trochlea
In 90° flexion	5. The superior part of the intercondylar notch, the Hoffa suspensory ligament 6. The intercondylar notch: femoral insertions of the ACL/PCL, posterior horns of the menisci 7. Tibial spine: tibial insertions of the ACL, the anterior horns of the menisci, intermeniscal ligament
In stressed valgus	8. The medial meniscus
Cabot position	9. The lateral meniscus and the popliteal tendon
In 30° flexion	10. The posteromedial compartment and posterior capsular attachment

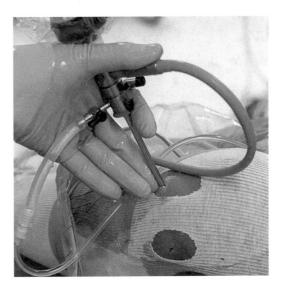

Fig. 1.16 The scope is being held by the middle finger against the skin and the thumb controls the light cable

Like in open surgery, the key to a successful operation is knowing how to hold the instruments. This is why we do not place our fingers in the forceps eyelets (Fig. 1.15). The hand and finger positioning should assure a better scope stability (Fig. 1.16).

In case of a difficulty in exposure, one of the first things to do is to cut the suspensory ligament of Hoffa to ensure a better vision (Figs. 1.17 and 1.18).

In order to visualize correctly the posterior horns, the light cable should be oriented upwards and the meniscus should be seen on a horizontal plane (Fig. 1.19).

A better view is obtained by a hip maneuver in extension that increases the valgus stress and offers a wider exposure.

The posterior horn of the menisci is tested with the hook probe in order to search for insta-

bility (dislocated under the femoral condyle) or a lesion.

The hook probe is passed under the meniscus and oriented upwards, at a 90° angulation, to unveil a hidden partial lesion (Fig. 1.20).

The posterior horn is better visualized by passing the scope in the intercondylar notch while aiming the light cable downwards (Figs. 1.21 and 1.22).

The ACL resistance to the hook probe is tested in the Cabot position allowing it to run over the femoral insertion (Fig. 1.23).

The passage into the posteromedial compartment is a part of the standard knee exploration.

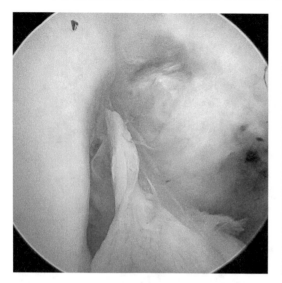

Fig. 1.17 The suspensory ligament of Hoffa

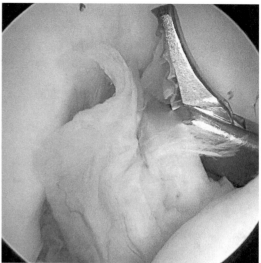

Fig. 1.18 Cut by a basket forceps

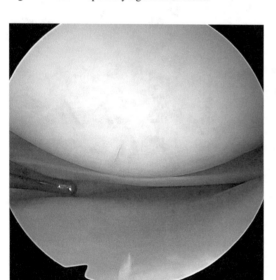

Fig. 1.19 The cable is oriented upwards

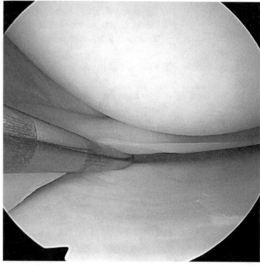

Fig. 1.20 Hook oriented upwards at a 90° angle to hold and uncover the hidden partial lesion

In order to do it, we have to pass in the space under the PCL and flush with the medial femoral condyle (Figs. 1.24, 1.25, and 1.26).

The crossing should be made with knee flexion from 0 to 30°. The foot is placed on the operator's pelvis with a free hand that could adjust the flexion to allow for the safe passage (Fig. 1.27).

Once the scope has passed into the posteromedial compartment, the knee is repositioned to a 90° angle of flexion and the exploration will be done only by adjusting the light cable since the scope will be stuck in the intercondylar notch (Fig. 1.28).

In this compartment, we can search for a posterior capsulomeniscal detachment called a ramp lesion. We should pay attention not to use the shaver while the aspiration is on at the risk of causing a lesion in the posterior capsule and especially the neurovascular elements close to the articulation while in extension.

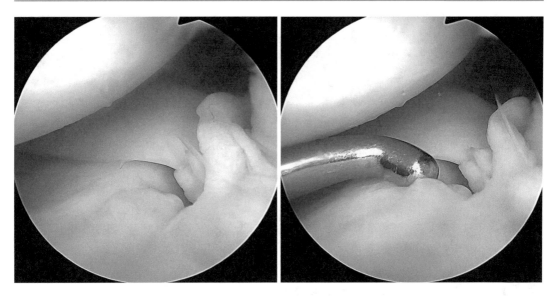

Figs. 1.21 and 1.22   A normal posterior horn, where a lesion is frequently associated with ACL ruptures

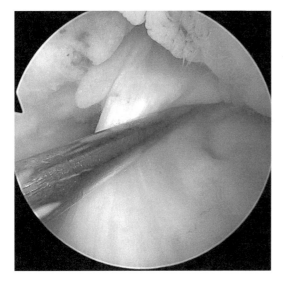

Fig. 1.23   Testing the ACL with the hook probe

In order to easily access the posterior horn of the meniscus, a "pie crusting" could be added with a needle in the posteromedial angle of the tibia, at the concavity curve level, a few centimeters below the articular line (Fig. 1.29). It aims at weakening the superficial fibers of the medial collateral ligament with the help of the needle. We should hear and feel crackles and see the opening of the compartment on the screen (Figs. 1.30 and 1.31).

Pain due to hematoma usually fades out in about 3 weeks without leaving any laxity.

The small bladed shaver is not systematically used but could be helpful especially in previous operated or synovitis-swollen knees.

The partial resection of the Hoffa's fat pad with a shaver in front of the anterior horns of the menisci helps better expose the different femorotibial compartments.

Even if the meniscal surgery tends to be the most conservative possible (abstention or sutures), the meniscectomy is still an important procedure in certain chronic conflict pain (positive grinding test on the physical exam) and for the non-suturable tears.

The meniscectomy is commenced using a basket forceps (Fig. 1.32) and smoothened by the shaver (Figs. 1.33 and 1.34).

Using angulated forceps and switching instrumental ports help us access difficult areas (Figs. 1.35 and 1.36).

When resecting a flap tear, be aware of losing the fragment once it is cut off from its neck. Fragments usually have a tendency to get stuck in the posterior compartment.

The meniscal fragments are evacuated by the trocar or aspirated with the shaver (Fig. 1.37).

At the end of the operation, the water is evacuated from the knee and the ports are closed with steri-strips (Fig. 1.38).

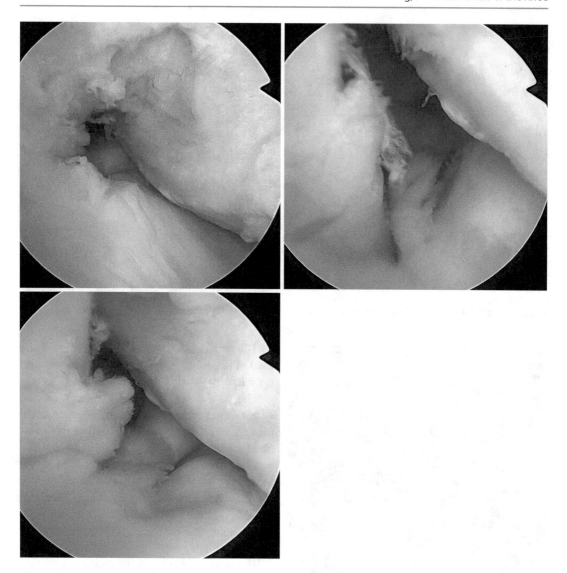

Figs. 1.24–1.26 Posteromedial passage

Fig. 1.27 The posteromedial crossing should be done progressively while adjusting the knee angulation between 0° and 30° of flexion

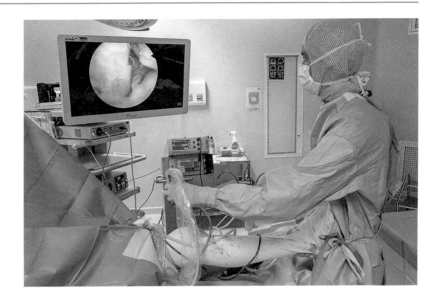

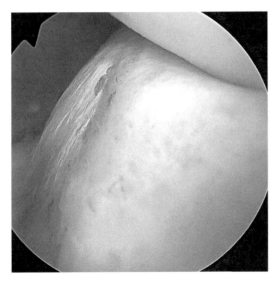

Fig. 1.28 A normal posterior capsulomeniscal attachment

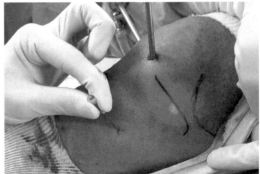

Fig. 1.29 Pie crusting is done a few centimeters below the articular line

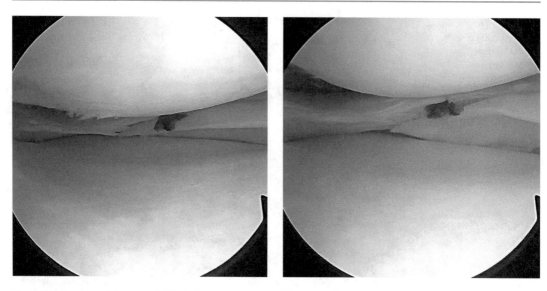

Fig. 1.30 Passage of the scope is blocked

Fig. 1.31 Opening of the compartment after pie crusting

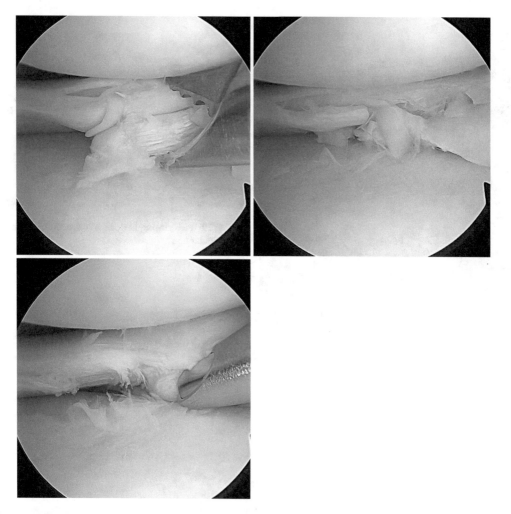

Figs. 1.32–1.34 Meniscectomy begun with a basket forceps and smoothened by the shaver

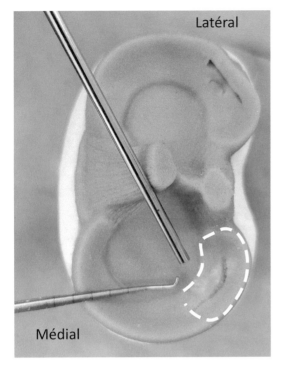

Fig. 1.35 Simple access to posterior horn

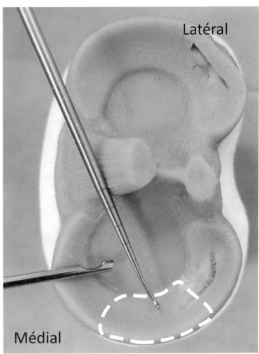

Fig. 1.36 Simple access to the middle horn after switching instruments

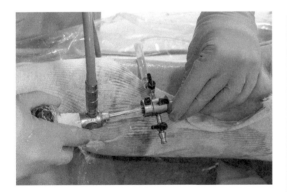

Fig. 1.37 The scope is detached from the trocar in order to evacuate the meniscal fragments

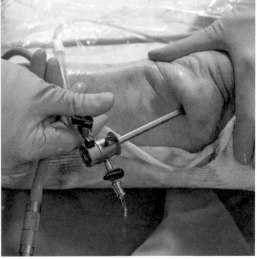

Fig. 1.38 Evacuating residual water from the trocar

Take Home Messages
- Make yourself comfortable.
- Patient positioning, cutting the Hoffa ligament, pie crusting, etc.
- Anticipate the location of the lesions in order to choose the right position of the ports.
- "Primum non nocere."
- Beware not to cause any iatrogenic damage to the cartilage tissue while forcing the instruments.

Meniscal Sutures: All-Inside, Out-In, and Posterior Horn Reinsertion

2.1 Overview

In meniscal surgery, the preoperative analysis of a tear on the MRI is essential.

It allows:

- The evaluation of its reparability weighing the factors of success versus the failure factors.
- The anticipation of the possible repair act and the prediction of its necessary material.
- The knowledge of a suspected tear in a specified location, so we will not miss it inadvertently.

In order not to forget anything, we have to be systematic and analyze the MRI on the three planes: sagittal, coronal, and axial planes.

In this example, the preoperative analysis of the MRI (Figs. 2.1, 2.2, 2.3, and 2.4) allows the planification of the bucket handle repair that extends into the anterior and middle horns (Figs. 2.5 and 2.6) before the ACL reconstruction, so we can have in place all types of meniscal sutures material for all techniques including all-inside and out-in repair.

2.1.1 The Abrasion

The first step of every suture technique is the abrasion of the two edges of the meniscus. We

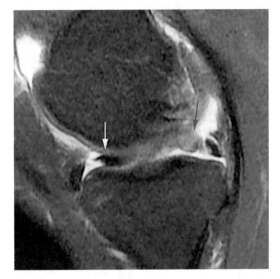

Fig. 2.1 In white, a double anterior horn aspect, in red truncated posterior horn

can use the shaver (Fig. 2.7), a diamond rasp (Figs. 2.8 and 2.9), or needles used in lumbar spine puncture (Fig. 2.10), in order to put in contact vascularized tissue on both edges of the tear.

2.1.2 The All-Inside Suture

The all-inside technique has the advantage of being simpler and faster than the others. It easily permits the stabilization of posterior and middle third-posterior third junction types.

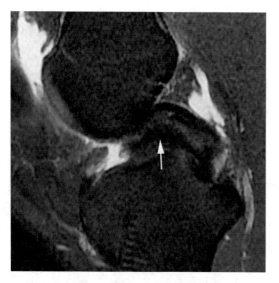

Fig. 2.2 In white, double PCL aspect

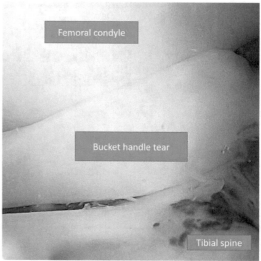

Fig. 2.5 A bucket handle tear dislocated in the condylar notch

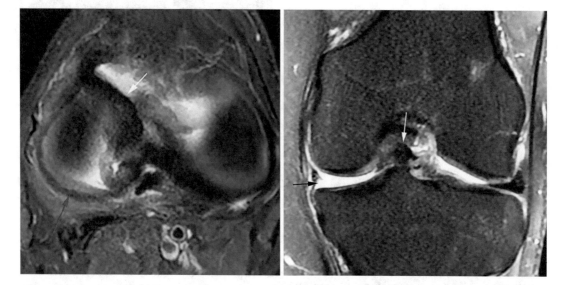

Figs. 2.3 and 2.4 A bucket handle dislocated into the condylar notch. In red, remaining posterior wall. In black, disappearing of the meniscus body

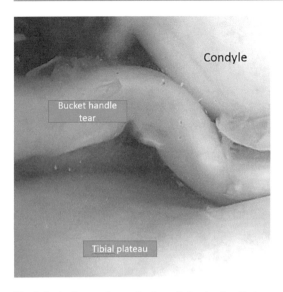

Fig. 2.6 An incomplete reduction of a bucket handle tear in the medial compartment

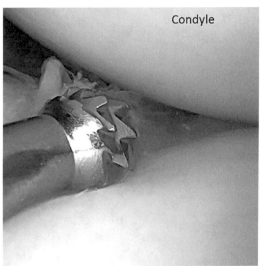

Fig. 2.8 Posterior abrasion

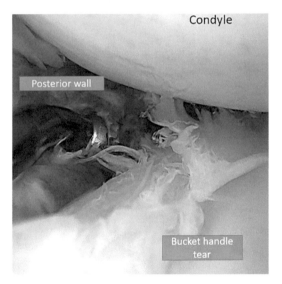

Fig. 2.7 Using a shaver

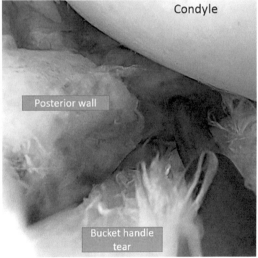

Fig. 2.9 Using a rasp

The needle length should be adjusted to 18 mm.

The semi-rigid and slightly fragile aspect of the system imposes:

- The utilization of an intra-articular guide/cannula, like a ramp, while the assistant holds the camera.

- Being perpendicular to the direction of the tear and maybe reversing the instrumental portal with the scope one.

A 5 mm space between sutures will ensure a rigid fixation.

This system helps us do all sorts of sutures adapted to the tear type: horizontal, vertical, or oblique.

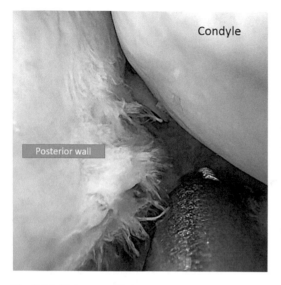

Fig. 2.10 Using a needle

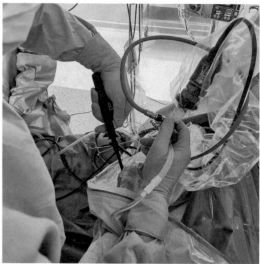

Fig. 2.12 All-inside technique system

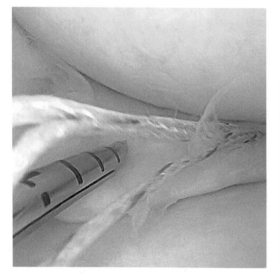

Fig. 2.11 Horizontal suture

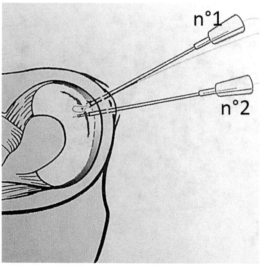

Fig. 2.13 Two-needle-out-in technique

The knot pusher is used to create tension on the suture to tighten it while avoiding direct traction on the wire and risk the tear of the fragile meniscus (Figs. 2.11 and 2.12).

2.1.3   Out-In Technique

Particularly used in the middle horn tears (body), it requires two needles (pink, 18G) and two PDS sutures.

The first needle is passed through the skin, with a wire loop inside, into the posterior wall while bridging the tear and then entering the joint.

An empty second needle is inserted in the same way, a few millimeters aside from the first one. A PDS suture is passed through this one (Fig. 2.13). Then the loop and the suture are passed through the instrumental portal with a grasping forceps (Figs. 2.14, 2.15, and 2.16).

The simple suture is introduced into the loop. This can be done both inside and outside of the knee (Fig. 2.17).

Then we pull in the two free strands in order to recover the simple suture and do the U suture (Fig. 2.18).

A small incision is made between the two entry points of the two needles (Fig. 2.19) in which the strands are recovered subcutaneously with a hook probe (Fig. 2.20). A simple knot is then made and will be applied to the capsule.

On the MRI, the tears on the roots associate radial tears (Figs. 2.21, 2.22, and 2.23) with meniscal extrusion.

The tibial spine is the place to look for the native insertion of the avulsed meniscal roots. Thus, we should look for the insertion of the medial posterior root that is 10 mm in front of the medial tibial spine, and that of the lateral posterior root that is 5 mm medial to the lateral tibial spine.

The reinsertion is done with two loop sutures passed through the root (Fig. 2.24) with the help

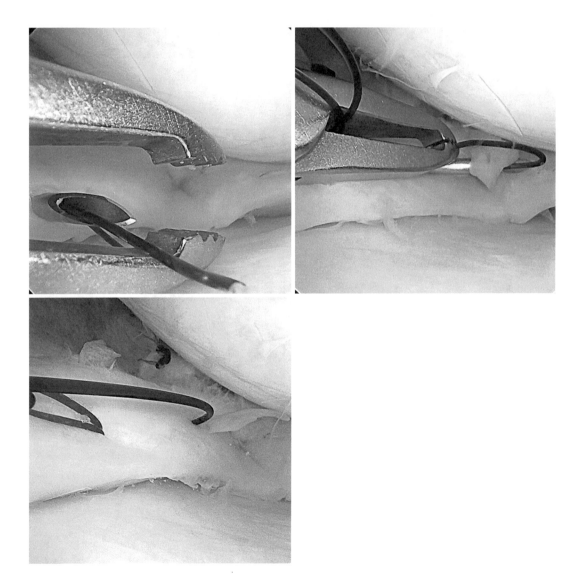

Figs. 2.14–2.16 A grasping forceps catches the loop and the suture in order to pass them through the instrumental port

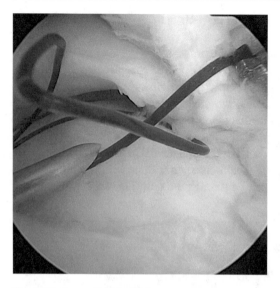

Fig. 2.17 Recovering the PDS suture

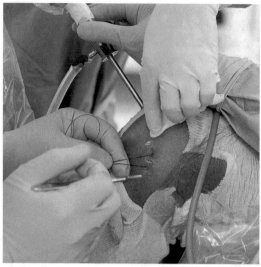

Fig. 2.19 Incision between the needles entry points

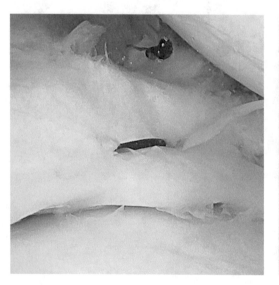

Fig. 2.18 U suture

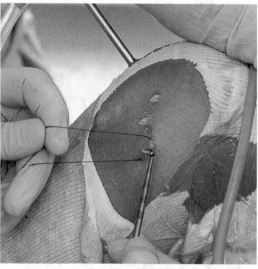

Fig. 2.20 A hook probe recovers the sutures and applies the knot to the capsule

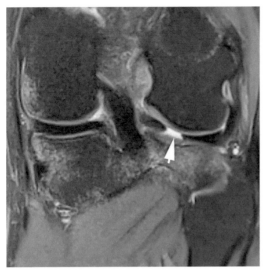

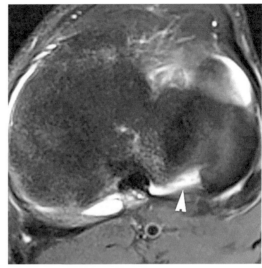

Fig. 2.21 Coronal vertical tear

Fig. 2.23 Perpendicular tear

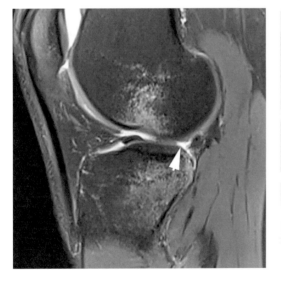

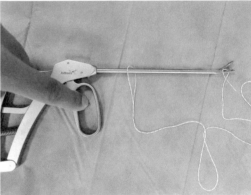

Fig. 2.24 A suture is passed through the root while aiming the condylar notch to avoid the condyle

Fig. 2.22 "Ghost" meniscus

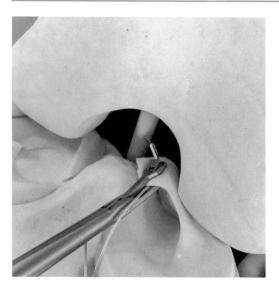

Fig. 2.25 A loop is previously fixed on the grasp forceps

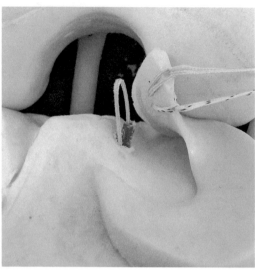

Fig. 2.27 The relay wire is recovered and unraveled with the other sutures

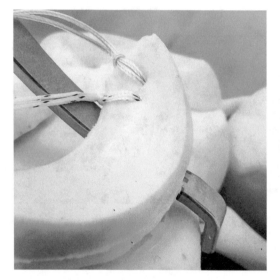

Fig. 2.26 The laser mark helps us precisely locate the emergence of the tunnel

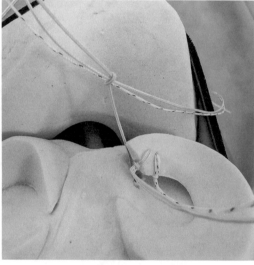

Fig. 2.28 With the relay wire, we pass the sutures exteriorly

of a rotator cuff grasper used in shoulder arthroscopy (Fig. 2.25).

A 3.5 mm tunnel is made with a special guide passed under the femoral condyle (Fig. 2.26). A relay wire is passed through the tunnel with a stick (Fig. 2.27). After they are unraveled, the sutures are passed through the tunnel using the relay wire (Fig. 2.28). The fixation to the cortical bone is done either by a screw or an endobutton (Fig. 2.29).

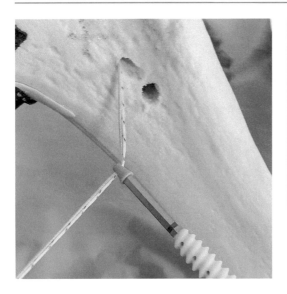

Fig. 2.29 The sutures are recovered and fixed

Take Home Messages
- The preoperative analysis of the tears and lesions is essential to anticipate the problems and material needed for the operation.
- The abrasion is an essential time for the healing process of the meniscus.
- Every suture has its specificity and characteristics. This is why we should be acquainted with all the techniques.

The Hamstring Graft: ACL Reconstruction with Quadruple Bundle Gracilis and Semitendinosus Tendons

3

3.1 Overview

The hamstring tendon graft reconstruction of the ACL is the most popular first intention procedure due to its simplicity and lesser morbidity related to graft harvesting. Harvesting seems to be the most delicate time of the procedure, forcing the surgeon to change tactics in case of failure.

Newest techniques involve the rapid "ligamentization" while preserving the tendons attached to their distal insertion on the tibia and keeping a maximum tissue of the native ACL while passing the graft through the stump.

One particular care is the positioning of the femoral tunnel in an isometric zone of the ACL's anteromedial bundle, behind the "resident's ridge," in order not to position it anteriorly, risking a postoperative flessum (flexion) and its failure.

3.2 Hamstring Tendons Graft Harvesting: Anterior Approach

The time dedicated to this harvesting is crucial. The quality of the graft dictates the success of the reconstruction.

The patient positioning is the same as used in knee arthroscopy at 90° angle of flexion with the use of a knee stabilizer and a stress post.

A short vertical or horizontal incision is made 3 cm under the knee joint line and medially to the tibial tuberosity (Figs. 3.1 and 3.2). Palpation helps rolling the tendons of the pes anserinus under our fingers in order to locate them. This sensation can be amplified while humidifying the fingers with a betadine solution.

The fat dissection is done with the help of the rugine of Lambotte in order to expose the pes anserinus' distal insertion on the tibia formed by the Sartorius, the gracilis, and the semitendinosus tendons (Figs. 3.3 and 3.4).

We make then a horizontal opening in the Sartorius tendon and "the hole" will appear (Fig. 3.5): a dissection space between the pes anserinus superficially and the medial collateral ligament deeply.

Under the Sartorius tendon, in the space we have created, we locate from top to bottom, the gracilis and then semitendinosus (Fig. 3.6). We are sure that we are in the right place!

The gracilis is externalized with the aid of a small dissector while grabbing it from its base. Then is carefully dissected from its inferior vincula (Fig. 3.7), the scissors oriented downwards while sliding through the tendon without forcing (Fig. 3.8), and paying attention not to damage it. When the tendon is more exteriorized, then we are sure to have sectioned all of the vincula.

To externalize and to facilitate its harvesting with the stripper, we need to:

- Replace the dissector with the finger (Fig. 3.9).
- Flex the knee to 120°.

O. Courage et al., *Knee Arthroscopy*, https://doi.org/10.1007/978-3-030-82830-1_3

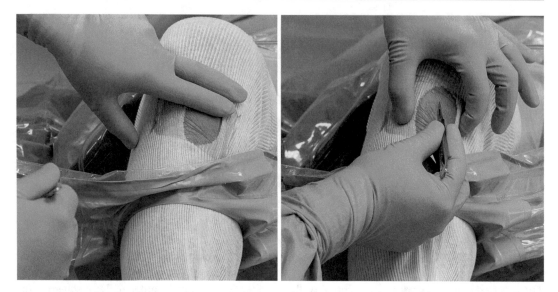

Figs. 3.1 and 3.2 A vertical incision made 3 cm under the knee joint line and 3 cm medially to the tibial tuberosity

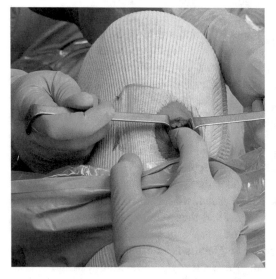

Fig. 3.3 Tracking the hamstring tendons with the finger

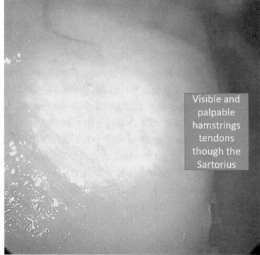

Visible and palpable hamstrings tendons though the Sartorius

Fig. 3.4 Tracking the hamstring tendons with the naked eye

We put the stripper in place and the gracilis is stripped while aiming towards the pubis (Fig. 3.10). This orientation helps decrease the efforts and lower the risk of tearing the graft.

In the same manner, the semitendinosus tendon is dissected and exteriorized. We aim this time towards the ischium, slightly more laterally, in order to be in the direction of the muscular body (Fig. 3.11).

The graft preparation is quick and simple. We begin by taking off the muscular part that is adherent to the tendon then fixing each bundle with a capstan knot using an absorbable suture maintained with several half hitch knots (Fig. 3.12).

The calibration of the tendons can be done despite the knot; usually, a 9 mm diameter is used (Fig. 3.13). Then they are left attached (Fig. 3.14),

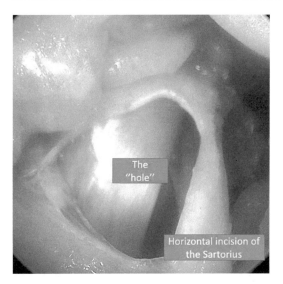

Fig. 3.5 "The hole," dissection space

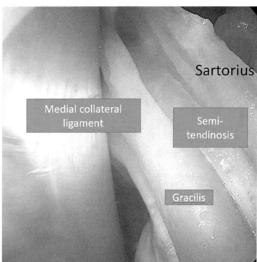

Fig. 3.6 Between the MCL on one side and the Sartorius on another

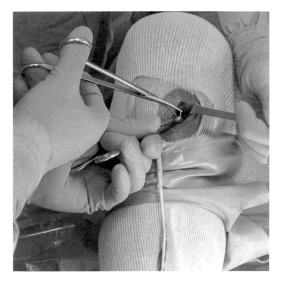

Fig. 3.7 The scissors help section the vincula

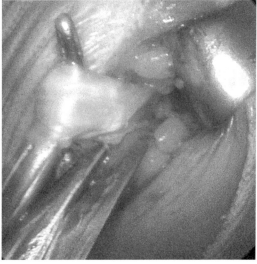

Fig. 3.8 Blades of the scissors pointed downwards to avoid damaging the graft

no measure is necessary at this moment, and both bundles are placed in the medial approach taking into consideration not to block the tibial guide.

3.3 Femoral Tunnel: First Part

We use two portals, one anterolateral and another anteromedial a little bit lower than the other, used for instrumentation (Figs. 3.15 and 3.16). The lat-

ter should be big enough to pass a 9 mm drill without damaging the skin.

The first part of the exploration consists of being sure of the absence of the "bell clapper" formation at the tibial insertion of the ACL (Fig. 3.17). Beside an anterior position, these formations can be partially hidden behind the Hoffa suspensory ligament. The flexion position helps

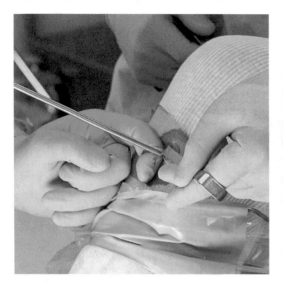

Fig. 3.9 The finger is placed around the graft to oppose the force of the stripper without pulling so hard on it

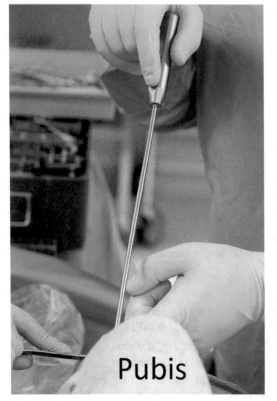

Fig. 3.10 For the gracilis, aim the stripper towards the pubis

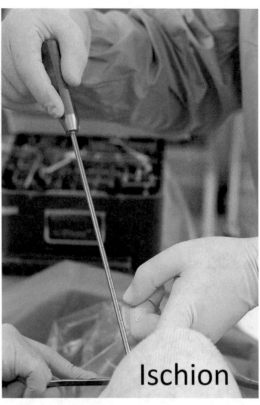

Fig. 3.11 For the semitendinosus, aim the stripper towards the ischium

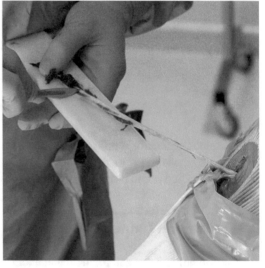

Fig. 3.12 With the help of a tilted blade, we remove the adherent muscle fibers

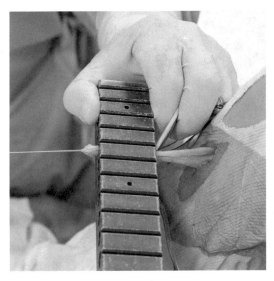

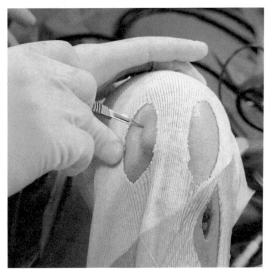

Fig. 3.13 Measuring the diameter with a knot attached to it

Fig. 3.15 Lateral port close to the patellar tendon

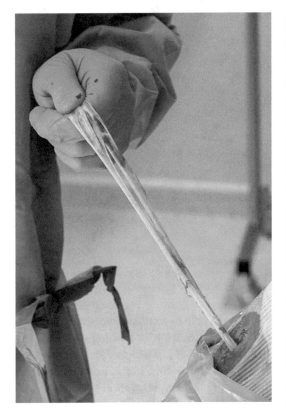

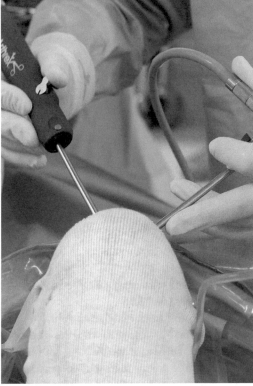

Fig. 3.14 Tendons left attached

Fig. 3.16 Triangulation

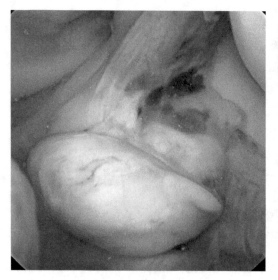

Fig. 3.17 Bell clapper formation

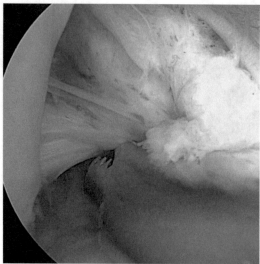

Fig. 3.19 The shaver is oriented towards the ACL residue

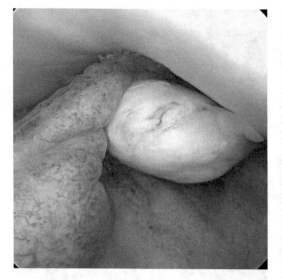

Fig. 3.18 Intercondylar notch conflict during extension

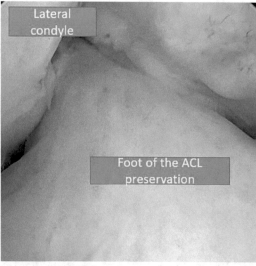

Fig. 3.20 We have to keep as much as native ACL as we can, in order to help "ligamentization" process

discovering and avoiding an anterior conflict postoperatively (Fig. 3.18).

We begin the intercondylar cleaning by sectioning the Hoffa ligament with the use of a shaver, then the rest of the ACL at its femoral insertion, while taking care not to section the PCL nor the footprint of the ACL (Figs. 3.19 and 3.20).

The access to the intercondylar notch is facilitated by the Cabot position.

With the help of a curette, we locate the "resident's ridge," the anterior limiting we should not surpass (Fig. 3.21). Then we place the curette behind this limitation, 5 mm in front of the posterior wall of the condyle, at an 11 o'clock orientation for the right knee and 1 o'clock for the left (Fig. 3.22).

In order to make a femoral tunnel, we do not use a femoral guide but an angled microfracture

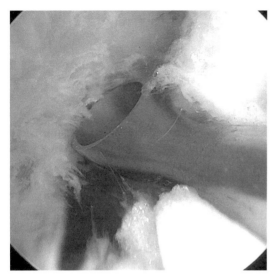

Fig. 3.21 Abrasion of the zone behind the resident's ridge

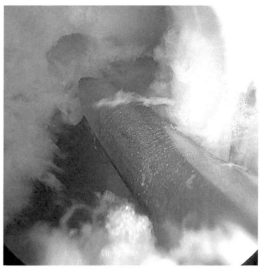

Fig. 3.23 Precise femoral tunnel with the help of an angled AWL

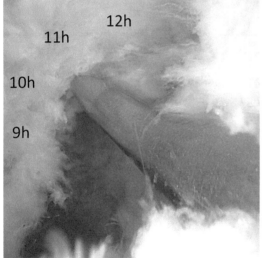

Fig. 3.22 We aim at an 11 o'clock orientation

Fig. 3.24 Verification of a presence of a posterior wall with a hook probe, behind the entry point of the femoral tunnel

AWL, used for Pridie microperforations (Fig. 3.23). In fact, the use of a guide has a disadvantage of letting soft tissue incarcerated between the guide and the wall, having a posterior tunnel and risking the formation of a "half pipe" (a tunnel with no posterior wall).

With the hook probe, we confirm the right position of the femoral tunnel (Fig. 3.24). At this moment, we conduct the knee exploration in search of a meniscal tear and a meniscal repair if possible.

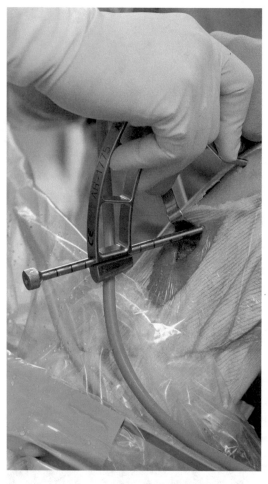

Fig. 3.25 Tibial guide firmly applied to the tibia

3.4   Tibial Tunnel

We place the tibial guide, in the easiest position, at the center of the native ACL stump that we left on purpose (Fig. 3.25).

The position should be the most posterior possible in order not to create a conflict with the intercondylar notch in extension, without reaching the internal tibial plateau so as to have a better obliquity of the new ACL and a better rotational control (Figs. 3.26 and 3.27).

A simple trick is to fix the K-wire at the top of the intercondylar notch, so the wire will not follow the drill once we remove it (Fig. 3.28).

We can now proceed with the drilling, beginning with the 6 mm drill and then pass directly to the final diameter, so we will not damage the native ACL stump (Fig. 3.29).

The tissue of the footprint of the ACL is preserved; this will help us keep living tissue around the graft.

3.5   Femoral Tunnel: Second Part

The femoral tunnel is made using the anteromedial post, in 120° of flexion.

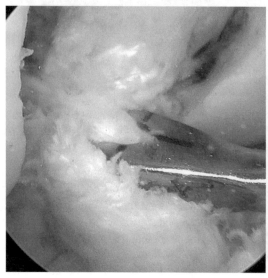
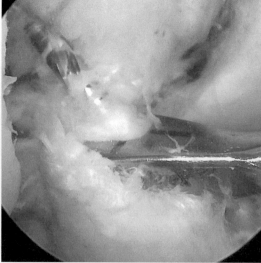

Figs. 3.26 and 3.27 At the footprint of the native ACL

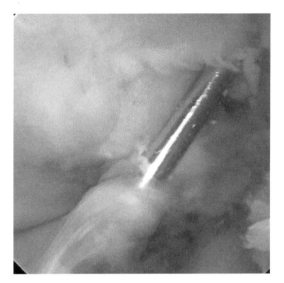

Fig. 3.28 The K-wire fixed at the intercondylar notch

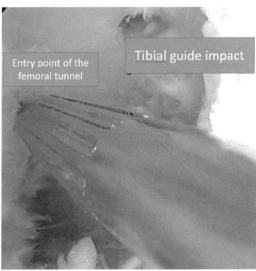

Fig. 3.30 Take care not to position the Beath pin at the entry point of the K-wire

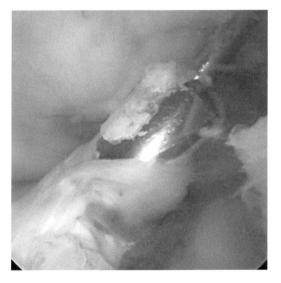

Fig. 3.29 The drills are passing through the stump of the native ACL

It begins by positioning the Beath pin at the entry point of the femoral tunnel previously prepared (Fig. 3.30).

A partial tunnel of 25 mm long is made using the 9 mm drill (Fig. 3.31).

3.6 Ascent, Tension Adjustment, and Transplant Fixation

A FiberWire tractor is passed through the Beath pin. This pin is then retrieved by hand taking the two free strands of the wire.

The loop is retrieved from the tibial tunnel through a grasper forceps via the native ACL stump (Fig. 3.32).

In order to know where to place the loop on the graft, we have to measure the total length of the graft passage using a flexible K-wire passed from the tibial through the femoral tunnel (Figs. 3.33, 3.34, 3.35, and 3.36).

The distance is measured and then projected onto the graft; the femoral loop is positioned at that place (Figs. 3.37, 3.38, and 3.39).

Then the guide pin of the interference screw is passed through the anteromedial port passing

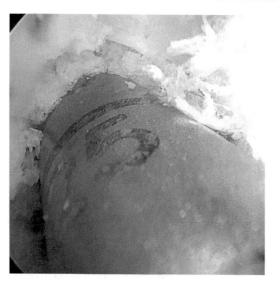

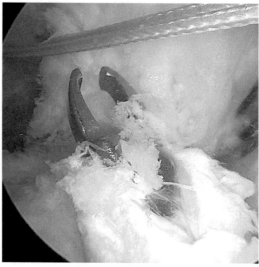

Fig. 3.31 A partial 25 mm long tunnel prepared with a 9 mm drill

Fig. 3.32 A grasper forceps helps retrieve the FiberWire through the stump

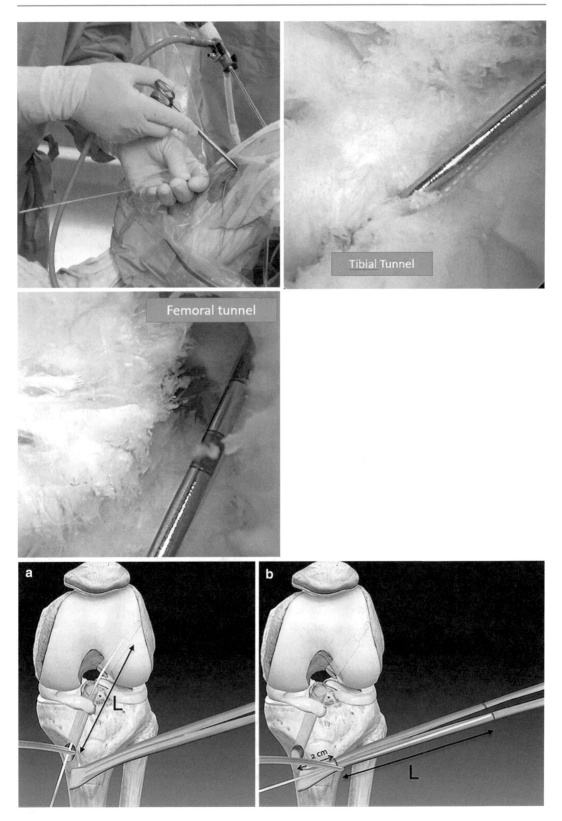

Figs. 3.33–3.36 K-wire insertion passed through the tibial into the femoral tunnel to measure the total length of the graft needed

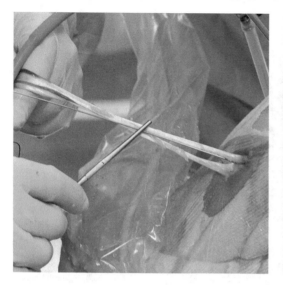

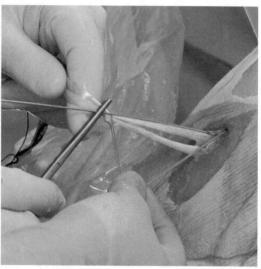

Fig. 3.37 The projection of the measured distance on the graft while adding the tibial tunnel distance-tibial insertion

Fig. 3.38 Loop positioning at the right distance

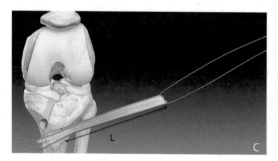

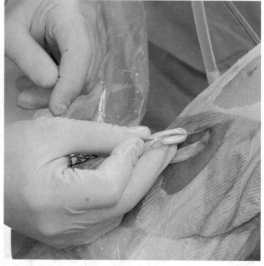

Fig. 3.39 The graft is folded at the right distance

through the femoral tunnel in order not to cause any conflict with the graft.

We can now proceed to the ascension of the graft that has been left attached in its distal part (Figs. 3.40, 3.41, 3.42, and 3.43).

Once the graft is well-positioned in the femoral tunnel with adjusted tension by the tractor wire, we fix the femoral part with a 7 mm interference screw. The fixation is done with the knee in flexion (Figs. 3.44 and 3.45). We have to make sure that the graft is well fixed while pulling the wires emerging from the tibial tunnel.

Fig. 3.40 The ascension of the graft, loop in place

We cycle the graft, and then we pass to the tibial fixation which is done in 20° flexion.

We place the guide pin in place, in front of the graft. Then we insert the 9.35 mm screw (Fig. 3.46). The hold is sufficient, no additional fixation is needed.

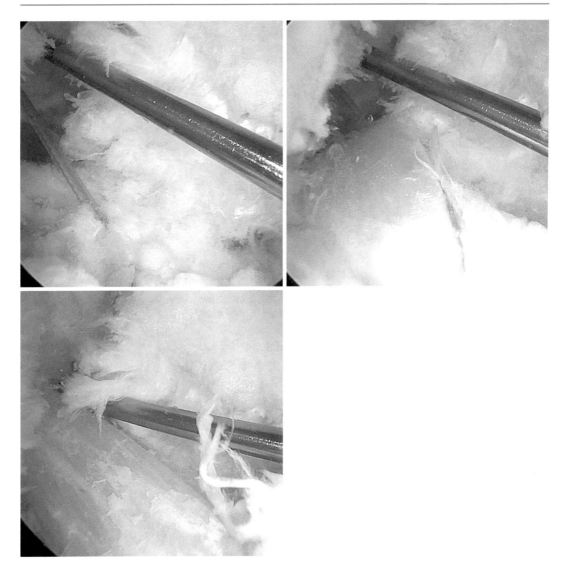

Figs. 3.41–3.43 The progressive ascension of the graft by continuous pulling with the femoral tractor wire. Note that the guide pin is inserted before the ascension

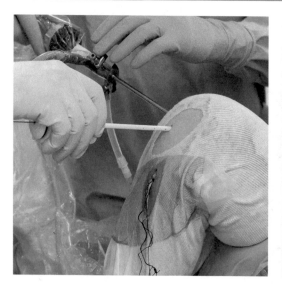

Fig. 3.44 Femoral fixation with an interference screw

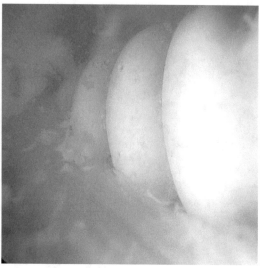

Fig. 3.45 Screw in contact with the graft, introduced in the femoral tunnel

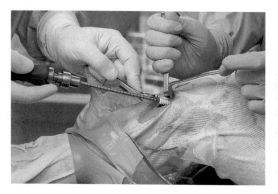

Fig. 3.46 Tibial fixation in slight flexion with an interference screw

We verify that the screw is sufficiently inserted into the tibial tunnel in order not to create a discomfort at the entry point (Figs. 3.47, 3.48, 3.49, and 3.50).

At the end of the intervention, we make sure that the graft is well fixed, there is not any conflict with the intercondylar notch, and that the graft is well oriented.

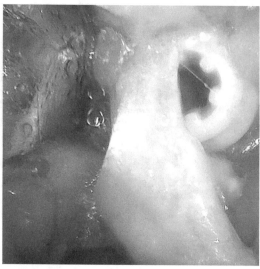

Fig. 3.47 An emerging screw from the tunnel that will potentially cause patient discomfort

The closure of the Sartorius is done and no suction drain is necessary.

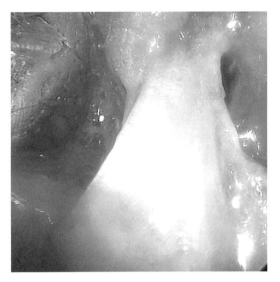

Fig. 3.48 A sufficient insertion of the screw

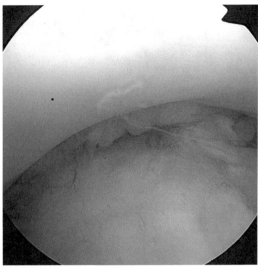

Fig. 3.49 Absence of conflict with the intercondylar notch

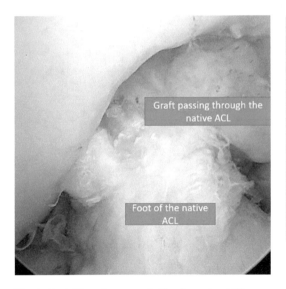

Graft passing through the native ACL

Foot of the native ACL

Fig. 3.50 ACL graft surrounded by the native ACL

Take Home Messages
- The time dedicated to graft harvesting is of paramount importance.
- The quality of the graft dictates the long-term results of the ACL reconstruction.
- The femoral fixation is a delicate time during an ACL reconstruction.
- We have to make sure the femoral tunnel is well-positioned.
- An anteriorly positioned femoral tunnel is the number one cause of ACL failure.

Quadruple Hamstring Graft: Single Four-Strand Semitendinosus Tendon

4.1 Overview

Different surgical techniques have been evolving over time to contribute to the creation of the use of a small graft.

First of all, the posterior approach hides the incision in the popliteal fossa, avoids the lesion of the branches of the saphenous nerve, and eliminates the risk of sectioning the transplant while stripping above the vincula. The use of a single hamstring tendon, the semitendinosis, as well as the use of a partial tunnel with a minimal incision ensure the mini-invasive characteristic of this technique.

Second, the use of the endobuttons for fixation is reliable, helps tensioning the graft, and is reproducible without secondary loosening.

Finally, the use of the out-in guide improves the femoral position precision avoiding any risk related to a crash of the posterior wall of the femoral tunnel.

4.2 Semitendinosus Tendon Harvesting Using the Posterior Popliteal Fossa Approach

The harvesting is done while having the knee at 30° of flexion maintained by the assistant.

The surgeon is positioned on the internal side of the knee while the assistant is on the external side (Fig. 4.1).

The semitendinosus tendon can be palpated under the skin at the medial third of the popliteal fossa. The incision is made 1.5 cm long, in the popliteal crease, yet the skin is slightly shifted medially to avoid sectioning the tendon (Figs. 4.2 and 4.3).

The bigger and more medially situated tendon is the semitendinosus. The fascia is incised medially to the tendon and 1 cm longitudinally and then dissected with the help of the right angle dissector to expose it and then tract it (Figs. 4.4, 4.5, 4.6, and 4.7).

The assistant places the leg on the table.

A loop tractor suture is passed around the tendon after clearing the fatting tissue on the tendon with a compress.

The association of the traction with the 90° flexion of the knee helps extrude the tendon (Figs. 4.8, 4.9, and 4.10).

An open stripper is used to free the tendon from its myotendinosis junction (Fig. 4.11a).

In the proximal part, there are no adherences. Thus, there is no risk of an early section of the tendon (Fig. 4.11b).

On the distal part, the harvesting is done with a closed stripper. It is performed by rotational movements of the wrist (without a significant traction on the tendon). This helps release the tendon from its distal adherences.

The detachment is made with the stripper while pulling the tendon in the direction of its fibers (Figs. 4.12 and 4.13).

© The Author(s), under exclusive license to Springer Nature Switzerland AG 2021
O. Courage et al., *Knee Arthroscopy*, https://doi.org/10.1007/978-3-030-82830-1_4

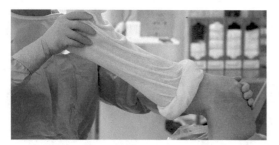

Fig. 4.1 During the incision and the dissection, the assistant maintains the knee flexed at 60°

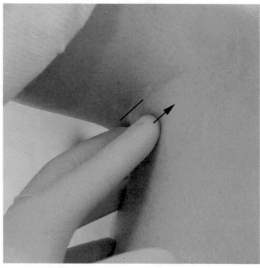

Fig. 4.3 1.5 cm incision, medially shifted

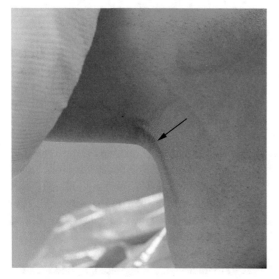

Fig. 4.2 The semitendinosus tendon

4.3   Graft Preparation

Graft preparation is done on the operating table, on a station dedicated to the continuous tensioning of the graft.

The first part consists of taking off all of the remainder of the vincula using a scalpel blade. To facilitate the procedure, the assistant holds the

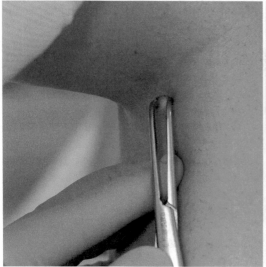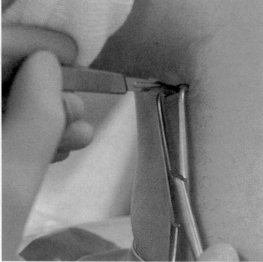

Figs. 4.4 and 4.5 Fascia exposed and incision with a scalpel no. 11

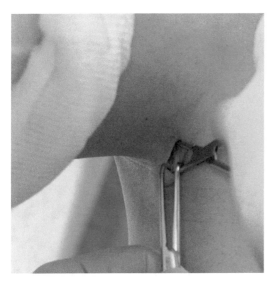

Fig. 4.6 Dissection with the right angle

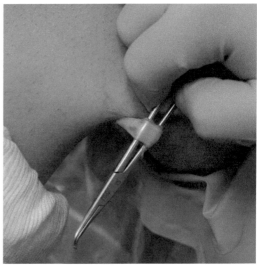

Fig. 4.7 Tendon extrusion

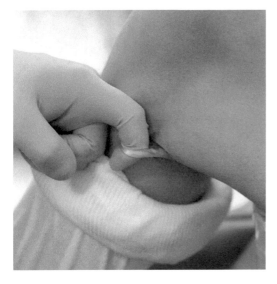

Fig. 4.8 Exteriorization of the tendon with the finger at 90 ° of flexion

graft at its two ends with two Kocher forceps (Figs. 4.14 and 4.15).

The second part of the preparation is the distance adjustment between the two hooks of the station at 60 mm. The minimal desirable length of the graft is:

- 30 mm corresponding to the intra-articular length.
- 15 mm in both the tibial and femoral tunnels (Figs. 4.16 and 4.17).

The third part consists of suturing the graft at its two extremities. A single whipstitch suture is made on the femoral end and two separate whipstitch sutures on the tibial side in order to obtain a homogenous tension on the four strands. The detailed technique shall be explained later on (Figs. 4.18, 4.19, and 4.20).

Once the graft is ready, its diameter is measured in order to know that of the tunnels. We choose the same diameter for the tunnel and the graft using the flip cutter so as to have a circumferential integration of the graft.

The last step is the tensioning of the graft. The tension is measured at 10 kg on the dynamometer. After continuous tensioning of the graft for about 15 min, a 5 mm stretching is seen. This pretensioning seems to reduce the secondary loosening of the graft.

During the arthroscopic tunnel preparation, the graft is covered by a humid compress.

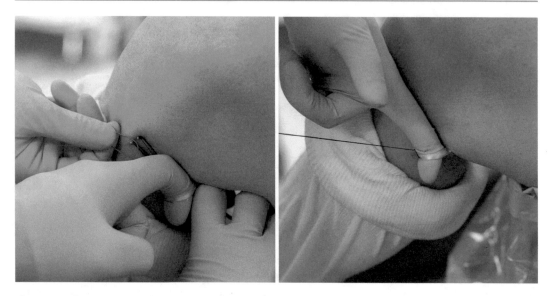

Figs. 4.9 and 4.10 Inserting the loop tractor wire

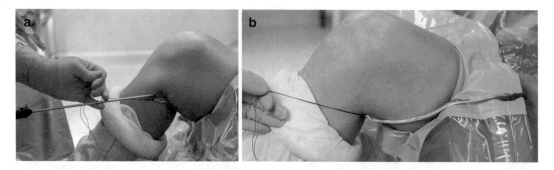

Fig. 4.11 (**a**) Stripping the tendon. (**b**) The semitendinosus is detached proximally

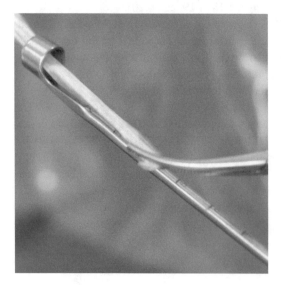

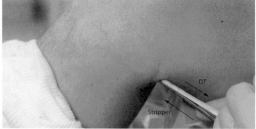

Fig. 4.13 Harvesting the distal part with a closed stripper to cut the vincula. The traction towards oneself is done only while detaching it from its insertion at the pes anserinus

Fig. 4.12 Tendon passed through the closed stripper

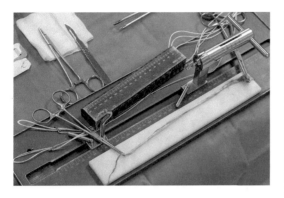

Fig. 4.14 Preparation on the table in a dedicated station

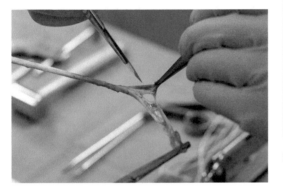

Fig. 4.15 Excision of the remainder of the vincula

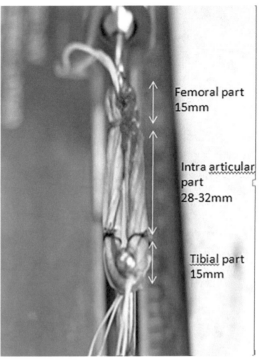

Femoral part 15mm

Intra articular part 28-32mm

Tibial part 15mm

Fig. 4.16 Length distribution throughout the graft

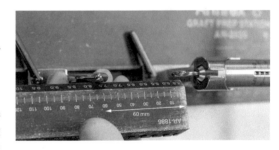

Fig. 4.17 The adjustment of the distance between the two hooks at 60 mm

4.4 Femoral Tunnel, Out-In Technique

A 15 mm tunnel is made with an out-in guide from the anterolateral port. During the learning curve period, it is recommended to drill a 20 mm tunnel to maintain a tension reserve.

The scope is handled by the assistant through the anteromedial port where the ACL footprint is better seen. The ACL native footprint is preserved to position the guide in its center. The femoral guide is adjusted at a 120° angulation. We have to be proximal to the epicondyle.

A cross-shaped incision is made on the fascia lata in the same direction of the guide, in order to let the endobutton pass through the fascia and to be anchored against the femoral bone (Figs. 4.21, 4.22, and 4.23).

The position of the femoral tunnel is at the center of the ACL footprint with the aid of the laser mark's guide while insisting on being posterior enough (Fig. 4.24).

The flipcutter, while closed, is introduced through the femur using the guide while waiting for its exit. The 180° rotation of the light cable helps us verify the complete opening of the flipcutter (Figs. 4.25 and 4.26).

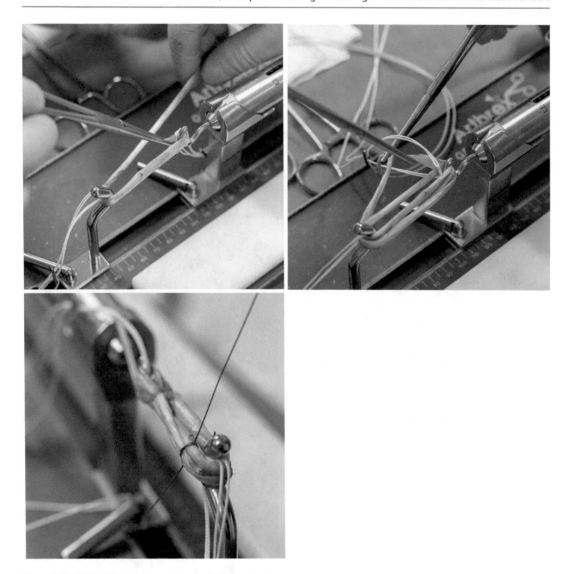

Figs. 4.18–4.20 Whipstitch technique of the semitendinosus

The aiming barrel of the drill guide is impacted onto the bone with a hammer. The rubber marker is pushed to reach the aiming barrel contact.

Reaming is begun at a maximal speed outside the cortical bone (to avoid breaking the reamer fin) without tearing the PCL, and then is prepared retrogradely.

Once the distance to the rubber band reaches 15 mm, we close the flipcutter and completely pull off the reamer.

Looped tracking wire is introduced through a plastic stick in the tunnel and recovered by the anteromedial portal with grasper forceps. The barrel is removed. The two ends of the tracking wire are put aside outside the knee (Figs. 4.27, 4.28, 4.29, and 4.30).

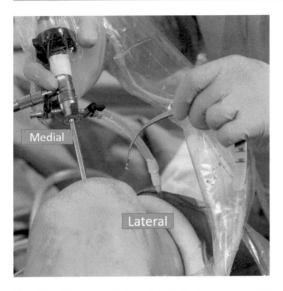

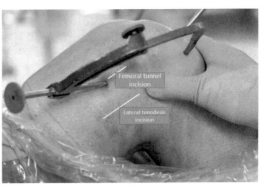

Fig. 4.23 The incision is at the level of the lateral femoral epicondyle that is palpated with the thumb. Be aware of the position of the lateral tenodesis incision that is posterior to the epicondyle

Fig. 4.21 The scope is introduced via the anteromedial port and the femoral guide is inserted into the anterolateral port

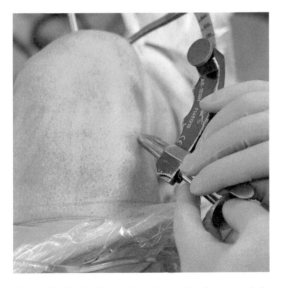

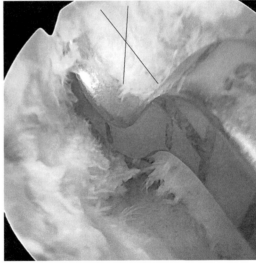

Fig. 4.22 The incision of the skin and the fascia lata is in the same direction as the femoral guide

Fig. 4.24 The footprint is at the center of the laser mark

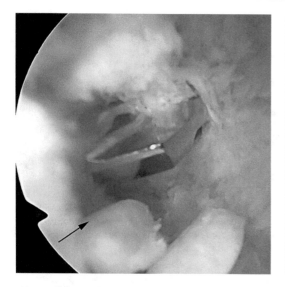

Fig. 4.25 The light cable in position to view the exit of the flipcutter

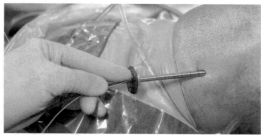

Fig. 4.27 The distance between the rubber and the aiming barrel

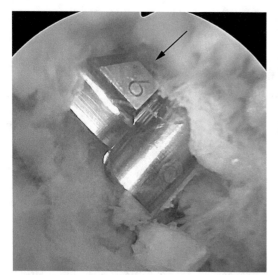

Fig. 4.26 The light cable turned 180° to make sure the flipcutter is fully opened

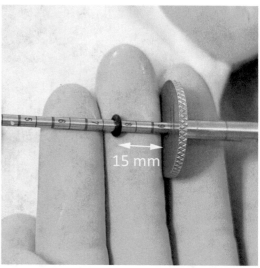

Fig. 4.28 The stick is introduced into the barrel with one end on the outside

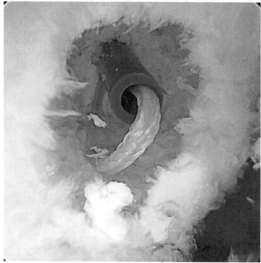

Fig. 4.29 A loop is then created in the knee

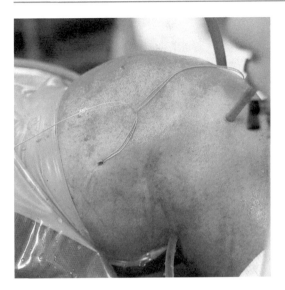

Fig. 4.30 The two free strands are passed through the loop and put aside

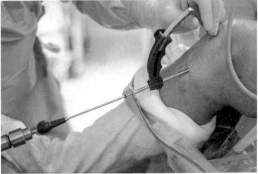

Fig. 4.31 Driving a tibial tunnel with a 70° angulation

4.5 Tibial Tunnel

Then we make the tibial tunnel in the same way.

The tibial guide is then adjusted to 70° of angulation and is positioned in a way that the entry point is halfway between the medial wall of the tibia and the ATT (Anterior Tibial Tuberosity). Here the hand is to be lowered: a tunnel that is more vertical than 70° ensures that the shape of the exit point is less oval and increases the precision of the position (Fig. 4.31).

Intra-articularly, the guide is positioned at the footprint of the native ACL. During the preparation, we preserve some of the native ACL tissue to ensure a better integration of the graft. The center of the footprint is removed with a shaver, where the guide is placed.

The closed reamer is then introduced. Once intra-articularly placed, the flipcutter is opened. Then at a maximal speed, we perform a retrograde reaming for a length of 25 mm. The tension reserve is privileged at the tibia where the osseous reconstruction is better than at the femur.

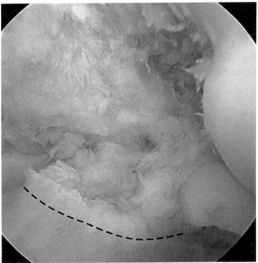

Fig. 4.32 Footprint of the native ACL

The last step consists of cleaning the intra-articular entry points of the tunnels with a shaver to facilitate the graft passage (Figs. 4.32, 4.33, and 4.34).

The loop of the tracking wire is different than the femoral one and is also introduced through a rigid plastic stick into the aiming barrel. We retrieve the loop through the anteromedial portal with a grasping forceps along with the femoral tracking wire to make sure that the two loops pass through the portal without the Hoffa fat pad interposition (Figs. 4.35, 4.36, and 4.37).

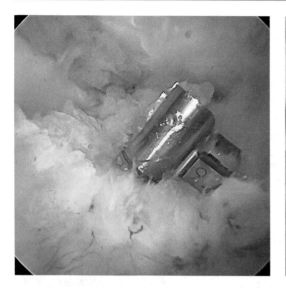

Fig. 4.33 Control of the complete opening of the flipcutter

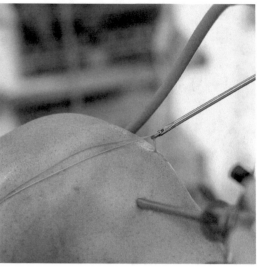

Fig. 4.35 The grasping forceps slides alongside the tracking wire

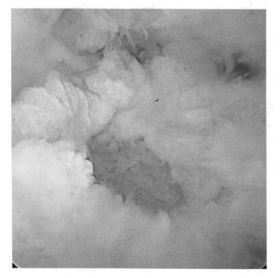

Fig. 4.34 Cleaning the entry point with a shaver

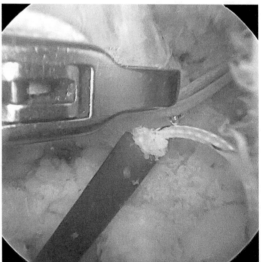

Fig. 4.36 Inside the knee joint avoiding Hoffa interposition

4.6   The Ascent, the Tension Adjustment, and Graft Fixation

The medial portal is extended with the Kocher forceps to enlarge the capsular opening for a smoother passage of the graft.

The strips of endobuttons are passed through the loop and the ascent is done progressively under visual control from the camera. Maintaining a certain tension will help the endobuttons progress in the same axis of the tracking wires at the entry point of the tunnel.

Once the endobutton passes the cortical bone, the resistance of the traction by the tibial strands confirms its impact on the bone. Before we cycle, we verify with the scope that it is introduced alongside the tracking wires and that there is no

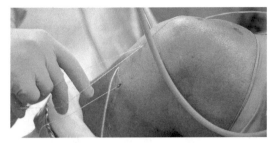

Fig. 4.37 Two loops are pulled off from the medial portal

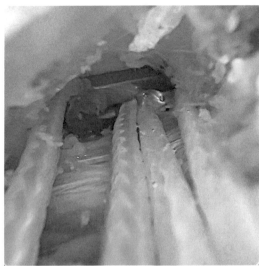

Fig. 4.39 The position of the endobuttons is verified while progressing the camera alongside the tracking wires, here completely impacted onto the bone

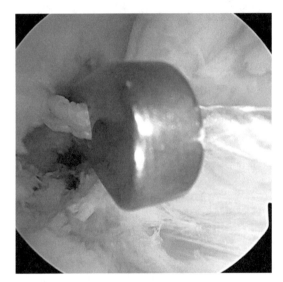

Fig. 4.38 Endobutton appearing at the same axis of the tunnel

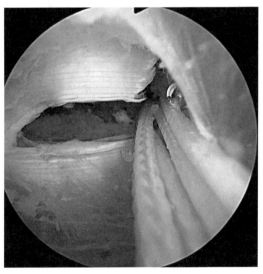

Fig. 4.40 While exiting the camera, we verify that there is no fascia lata interposition between the cortical bone and the endobuttons

interposition with the fascia lata (Figs. 4.38, 4.39, and 4.40).

We can now tighten the femoral endobutton for the first time while ascending the graft till the whipstitch mark (15 mm landmark from the extremity).

Now we introduce the tibial part with the help of its dedicated tracking wire. The button is placed at the entry point of the tunnel then exteriorized by tracting in one pull through the tibial tunnel medial approach.

Before tensioning the tibial part, the graft is exteriorized from the tibial tunnel till the landmark of the suture appears, using a hook, making sure that 15 mm of the graft is present in the tunnel. Then we complete the femoral tensioning, the femoral landmark is less visible during this step (Figs. 4.41, 4.42, and 4.43).

After cycling, the graft tensioning is finalized from each side in an extended position. A 30° flexion fixation risks postoperative flessum by overtensioning of the graft.

Using the scope, we finish by making sure the endobuttons are well positioned on the tibial and femoral bones.

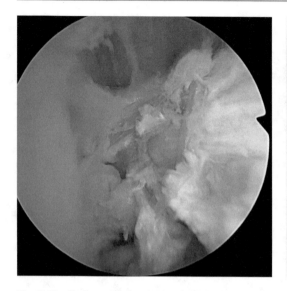

Fig. 4.41 Graft ascended to the femur till the landmark is reached

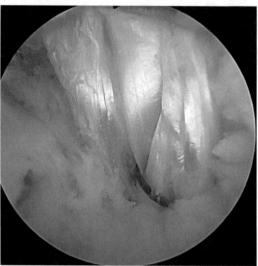

Fig. 4.43 We finish by impacting the endobutton onto the tibia. The suture landmark makes sure that 15 mm of the graft is made in each tunnel

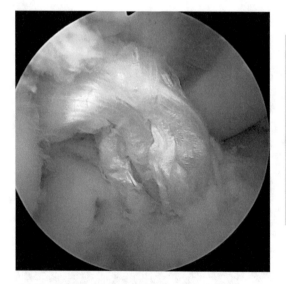

Fig. 4.42 The transplant is exteriorized from the tibial tunnel to finalize the femoral tensioning

Take Home Messages
- Mini-invasive technique: minimal scars, one hamstring tendon is harvested posteriorly, one-sided tunnel.
- Several traps and a demanding technique but easily reproducible if respecting each step.
- Precise tensioning but be aware of the balanced graft distribution in the two tunnels.

BTB Graft Technique: ACL Reconstruction Using the Patellar Tendon

5.1 Overview

The ACL reconstruction using the BTB graft, which was passed on to me by Bruno Locker, is old enough to gain a sufficient hindsight. Its longevity proves the reliability of the BTB fixation and its excellent results. This technique has not changed for the last 30 years.

We reserve it now for the redo cases after failure of the first ACL reconstruction using the hamstrings and exceptionally as a first intention treatment.

For the young surgeons who do not regularly use this technique, they will have a difficulty performing it in redo cases due to lack of automaticity and the presence of numerous pitfalls.

5.2 Patellar Tendon Harvesting

We prefer one unique anterior approach centered on the middle one-third of the tendon, starting from the apex with 7 cm distal stretch. This will ensure a better reliability of the tendinous graft.

The approach should be as little as possible while making sure that it is sufficiently extended distally in order to prevent a tibial tunnel that is too proximal or too short. In fact, the tibial tunnel will be made through the same approach.

Before doing the incision, we can evaluate the elasticity of the skin by mobilizing it around the patella in order not to extend the incision proximally (Figs. 5.1 and 5.2).

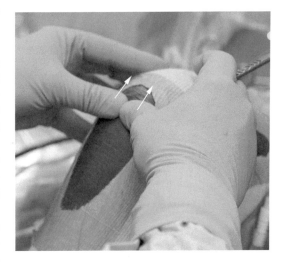

Fig. 5.1 Testing the skin elasticity

The pretendinous velum of the patellar tendon is opened carefully with the blade, reaching its borders in order to close it at the end of the procedure. Therefore, the patellar tendon is completely exposed.

The middle one-third of the tendon is cut, with a 9–10 mm diameter using two unique passages to avoid tendon delamination or one unique passage using the double bladed scalpel (Fig. 5.3).

Rather than fighting with the Farabeuf retractors, one trick is to expose the proximal part using the pointed bone reduction forceps positioned on the patella.

The outlines of the bone blocks can be drawn using the electrode blade following the lines on the tendon to facilitate the bony cuts (Fig. 5.4).

© The Author(s), under exclusive license to Springer Nature Switzerland AG 2021
O. Courage et al., *Knee Arthroscopy*, https://doi.org/10.1007/978-3-030-82830-1_5

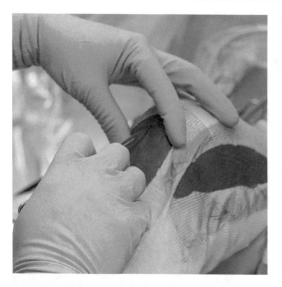

Fig. 5.2 Limiting the extent of the incision

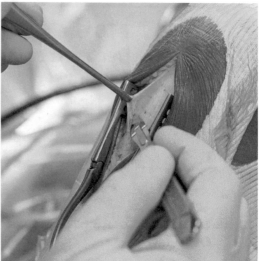

Fig. 5.3 Dissection of the pretendinous velum

The bony cuts are performed with a 45° inclination from bottom to top to obtain a trapezoidal patellar bony plug of 20 mm in length. A Farabeuf retractor protects the tendon from the oscillating blade.

The transverse cut is done twice, starting from each angle with a 45° inclination so it will not get stuck (Fig. 5.5).

Then we remove the patellar bony plug with an osteotome. To decrease the risk of fractures, we should be hearing the cracking sound of the cancellous bone before using the osteotome as a lever arm.

The dissection of the tendon should be done carefully. We should also dissect the Hoffa fat pad using the scissors without removing it from its insertion, so we will not complicate our arthroscopy procedure with water leakage (Figs. 5.6 and 5.7).

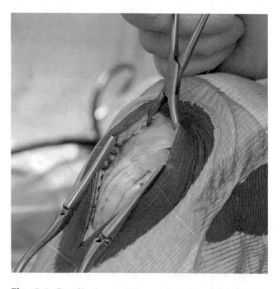

Fig. 5.4 Proximal exposition using the pointed bony forceps

Key Point: Detect the Tibial Insertion Height of the Tendon

Once the tendon is completely dissected, we can then easily locate the height of the tibial insertion making sure that we have sufficient tibial bone harvesting. One frequent error is to retrieve a small tibial bony plug while underestimating the real ATT insertion of the tendon. One trick, in that case, is to inverse the sides of the graft: the tibial side is used for the femoral tunnel and the patellar side is used for the tibial tunnel.

On the tibial part, we do the bony cuts in the same way we did on the patellar side but making sure we take a bigger plug: 11 mm large so it will press fit and 25 mm in length (Fig. 5.8).

We should always follow these steps in order to avoid the first pitfall which is the graft harvesting!

We give the tip of the patellar plug a warhead shape using the gouge forceps to facilitate its insertion in the femoral tunnel. It will be calibrated slightly less than 10 mm to a better ascent of the graft (Figs. 5.9 and 5.10).

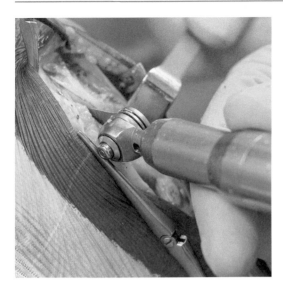

Fig. 5.5 A 45° inclination to harvest a trapezoidal bony plug

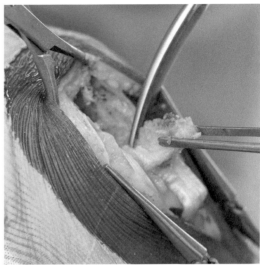

Fig. 5.7 Hoffa fat pad dissection from the patellar tendon

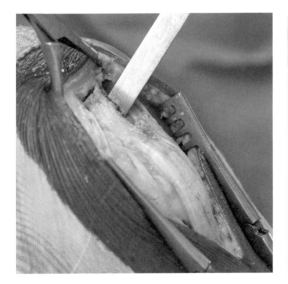

Fig. 5.6   Plug removal with the osteotome

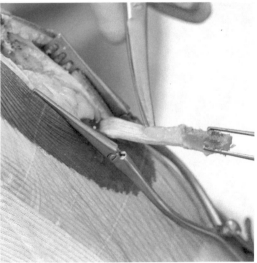

Fig. 5.8   Dissection of the ATT insertion

5.3   Preparing the Femoral Intercondylar Fossa

The scope is passed through the Gilquist port, in the middle of the Hoffa fat pad, while being as close as possible to the patella in order to be as high as possible.

The instrumental port is made through the median approach too (Figs. 5.11 and 5.12).

At first, we proceed to the clearing and cleaning of the intercondylar fossa like in all techniques.

In this case, we do not leave ACL remnants due to fear of conflict with the femoral bony plug of the graft. It is very important to clean the opening of the tunnels with the shaver to facilitate the ascent of the graft.

Like in the hamstrings graft harvesting technique, we use an angled microfracture awl with-

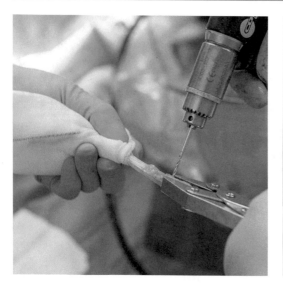

Fig. 5.9 1.5 mm diameter holes for the tracking wires to pass

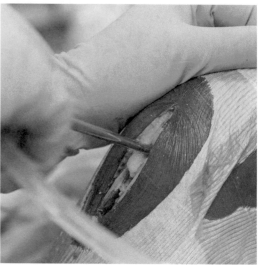

Fig. 5.11 Introduction in the middle of the Hoffa fat pad just below the patella

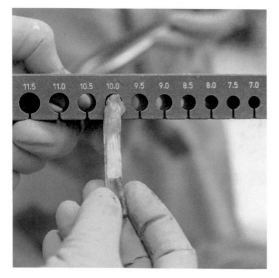

Fig. 5.10 Calibration of the bony plugs

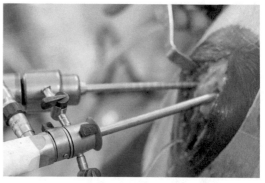

Fig. 5.12 Instrumental port through the same median incision

While the hook is in the correct position, we complete the meniscal exploration.

out a dedicated guide. This will help us do a marked hole, 5 mm anterior to the posterior wall of the femoral condyle.

For a right knee, it will be located at 11 o'clock, for a left at 1 o'clock. The position is checked with a hook probe to make sure that we are posterior enough (Figs. 5.13 and 5.14).

5.4   Tibial Tunnel

We begin with the tibial tunnel. We have to pay attention to the positioning of the tibial guide: at the intra-articular entry point and at the same time at the cortical entry point.

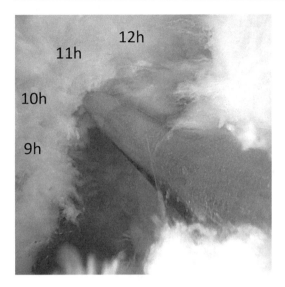

Fig. 5.13 Entry point of the femoral tunnel

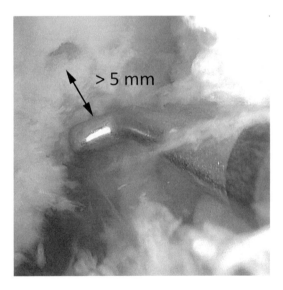

Fig. 5.14 Making sure that we have sufficient posterior wall thickness to reduce the risk of tunnel collapse

Intra-articularly, we aim for the ACL footprint while being slightly medial, paying attention not to damage the cartilage of the tibial plateau, and posterior to limit the conflict with the intercondylar notch. This position will ensure an obliquity that will offer a better rotator stability of the knee.

While positioning the guide on the cortical wall, we have to remember that the tibial tunnel has a minimum length of 35 mm (Figs. 5.15 and 5.16).

Once the guide pin is positioned on the desired place, we should collapse the cortical wall with a 10 mm auger.

The rest of the tunnel is done using a 10 mm trephine guided by a pin. We should pay attention while passing intra-articularly not to damage the condylar cartilage following the axis of the tunnel.

Once the bony plug is removed and placed aside for closure, a bone-tunnel-plug helps keep a sufficient intra-articular pressure (Fig. 5.17).

We can now clean the intercondylar fossa, but this time with a maximal flexed knee for the femoral tunnel, or by introducing the shaver via the tibial tunnel.

5.5   Femoral Tunnel

With the knee flexed at 120° and maintained by the assistant, we insert the trocar tip wire into the entry point.

Then we use the anteromedial port to drive the femoral tunnel with an auger of 10 mm large. It should be at least 25 mm in length to make sure that the tibial plug does not exceed the cortical wall.

We make sure that we have an intact posterior wall with the hook probe.

The suture is passed with the trocar tip pin, with the loop side left intra-articularly, and then retrieved by the tibial tunnel with the grasp forceps.

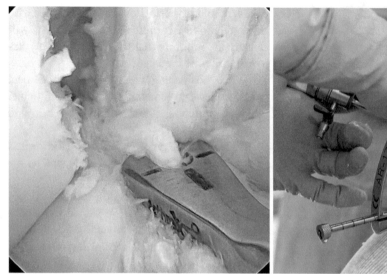

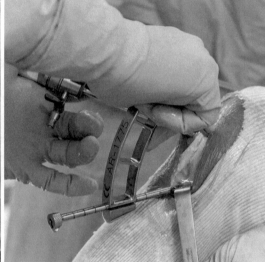

Figs. 5.15 and 5.16 Guide positioning on the ACL footprint

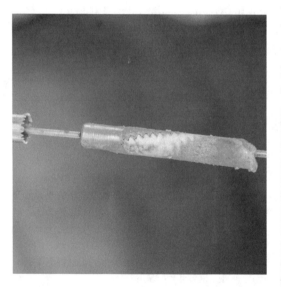

Fig. 5.17 A bony plug in a revision surgery: notice the screw inside the plug

5.6   Ascent, Tension Adjustment, and Transplant Fixation

Henceforth, we can ascend the graft (Figs. 5.18 and 5.19).

> **Key Point: Facilitate the Graft Ascent**
> The ascent of the bony plugs should be done with hard "frictions."
> In order to facilitate its ascent, we have to:
>
> - Aspirate all the residues with the shaver, especially in the tibial tunnel, particularly in redo cases (bone fragments, screws, and wires to extract).
> - Make sure that the entry point of the femoral tunnel and the exit point of the tibial tunnel are well freed from any debris, so nothing could affect the graft ascent.

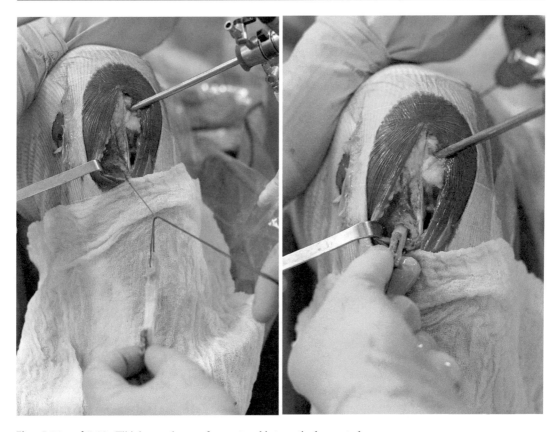

Figs. 5.18 and 5.19 Tibial transplant graft ascent and intra-articular control

The patellar plug will be inserted in the femoral tunnel with its cancellous part anteriorly and the ACL adherence on its posterior part. Therefore, we use the hook probe intra-articularly to orient the plug in front of the entry point of the tunnel.

We have to make sure not to have a "half pipe" phenomenon, with a tunnel too posterior causing a posterior wall collapse. In that case, it is difficult to fix the graft to the bone, and we should therefore drill another tunnel using the out-in technique with an endobutton fixation.

Then we insert the plug into the femoral tunnel (Fig. 5.20).

The guided pin is positioned anteriorly to the plug so that the interference screw will press back the plug to the bone.

We tap the femur. We make sure that the tibial plug will not pass beyond the tibial cortical wall

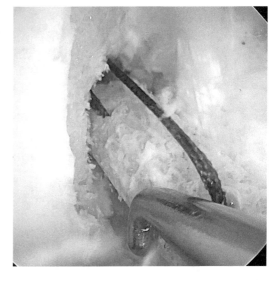

Fig. 5.20 The positioning of the plug is done with the help of the hook probe

and the intra-articular part. Then, while the assistant is maintaining a tension on the graft, we place a 7 mm diameter screw (Figs. 5.21 and 5.22).

Once the femoral fixation is complete, we have to always test its stability.

With the help of the scope, we insert the tibial guided pin anteriorly into the plug too.

Then we proceed to the fixation of the tibial screw while bending the knee to 20° of flexion, after cycling of the knee. Note that we do not tap the tibial entry point due to the cancellous nature of the tibia (Fig. 5.23).

Once fixed, we make sure that the screw is sufficiently inserted without passing the joint using the finger and the arthroscope (Figs. 5.24 and 5.25).

We make sure that there is no conflict between the foot of the graft and the intercondylar fossa in an extension position (Figs. 5.26 and 5.27).

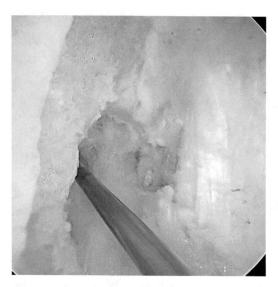

Fig. 5.21 Pin anteriorly positioned

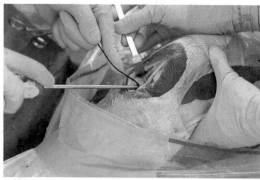

Fig. 5.23 While keeping tension on the graft, the surgeon fixates the screw in a near extension position

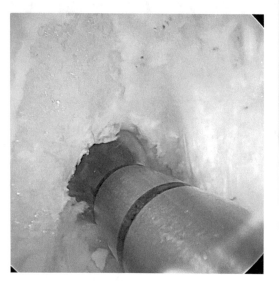

Fig. 5.22 Screw fixation holding back the plug

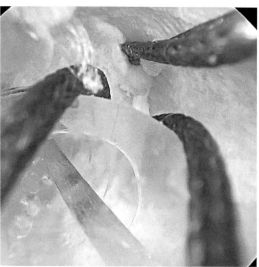

Fig. 5.24 Screw sufficiently inserted

5.7 Closure

Before closing the wound, we place the plugs we retrieved with the trephine, one at the patellar donor zone, and another on the tibial part. We can also use a cancellous allograft to fill the gaps (Figs. 5.28 and 5.29).

We do the combing of the patellar tendon then we close the pretendinous velum over the plugs we inserted (Fig. 5.30).

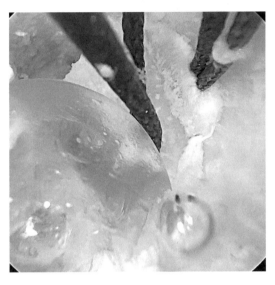

Fig. 5.25 Screw in position

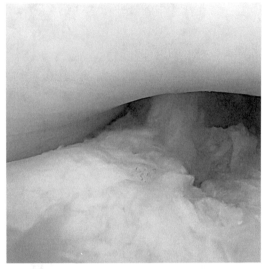

Fig. 5.27 Absence of conflict at extension

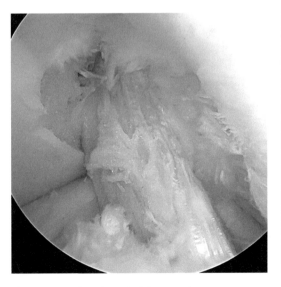

Fig. 5.26 Graft at the end of the operation

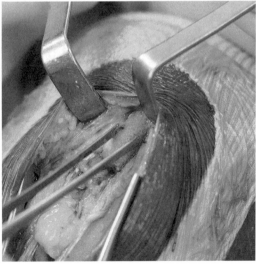

Fig. 5.28 Filling the donor patellar site

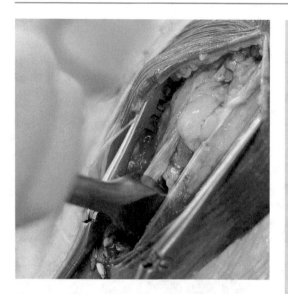

Fig. 5.29 Filling the tibial site with the cancellous plug

Take Home Messages
- Pay attention to the tibial insertion of the patellar tendon to the ATT to avoid harvesting a small graft.
- The weak point of the fixation is usually the femoral part.
- Always make sure you have sufficient posterior wall thickness on the femoral tunnel.
- The passage of the bony plugs should be through hard friction in the tunnels in contrary to the hamstrings graft technique.
- To help the ascent of the graft, we have to make sure that we cleaned the entry points enough.

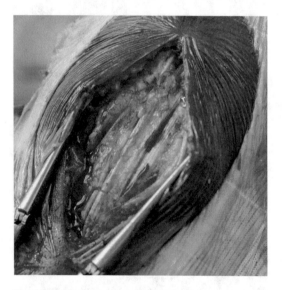

Fig. 5.30 Final combing of the tendon

Lateral Tenodesis: Extra-articular Reconstruction with the Fascia Lata Using a Modified Christel-Djian Technique

6

6.1 Overview

This tenodesis is an additional procedure to the ACL reconstruction.

It has a role in controlling rotational instability of the tibia while limiting the anterior translation of the lateral tibial plateau. Thus, it has a role in protecting the graft and contributes to controlling the pivot shift clunk.

Its indications are growing: pivot contact sports, explosive pivot shift tests, young patients, Segond fractures, medial meniscal tears, redos, increased tibial slope, etc.

6.2 Harvesting

We chose a simple technique that consists of retrieving a band of the fascia lata just cranially to the lateral femoral condyle.

The skin incision starts at the lateral epicondyle and extends 4 cm proximally in the direction of the fascia lata fibers (Fig. 6.1).

We retrieve an 8 mm large bundle and 5 cm in length that we leave attached distally (Fig. 6.2). The difference with the original technique is that our harvesting excludes its detachment on the Gerdy's tubercle.

The preparation of the graft ends with the making of a capstan knot at the proximal part using a tracking wire that will be inserted in the tunnel for a total length of 20 mm (Fig. 6.3).

6.3 Fixation

The goal is to make a complete circular tunnel:

- with sufficient length to place the graft at tension
- without crossing the femoral ACL tunnel

> **Key Point: Location the Femoral Fixation Entry Point**
>
> We locate the femoral fixation point, which is 5 mm posteriorly and 5 mm cranially to the external condylar tubercle.
>
> While dissecting to reach the point of entry, the presence of three arterioles that we will coagulate confirms the good positioning of the fixation.

A trocar tip pin is inserted and oriented upwards (directed towards the anteromedial cortex) while aiming the patellar base (Fig. 6.4).

Tapping is performed using a 6 mm diameter auger for a 30 mm length.

A relay wire is inserted in the tip of the pin while leaving the knot on the lateral side. The pin is then retrieved.

The graft is passed through the loop while folding it into two bundles allowing a much more solid fixation (Fig. 6.5).

© The Author(s), under exclusive license to Springer Nature Switzerland AG 2021
O. Courage et al., *Knee Arthroscopy*, https://doi.org/10.1007/978-3-030-82830-1_6

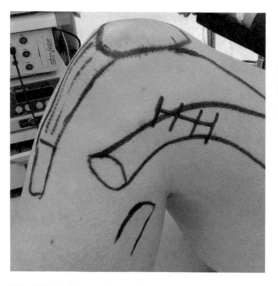

Fig. 6.1 Incision mark over the lateral epicondyle

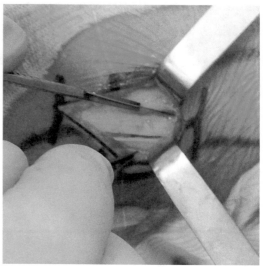

Fig. 6.3 An 8 × 50 mm bundle

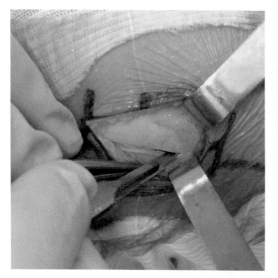

Fig. 6.2 Incision of the Fascia Lata

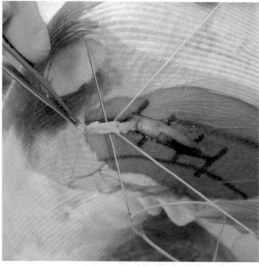

Fig. 6.4 Aiming over the patellar base

The guided pin of the fixation screw is inserted before we insert the graft into the tunnel.

The ascent of the graft is done while pulling the relay loop therefore helping to control perfectly its tension.

The screw is fixated while holding the knee at a near extension position (Fig. 6.6), foot in neutral position, to reduce external rotation restraint.

We use the same screw we use in the fixation of the Long biceps tendon.

It is to be noted that this technique is easy and that the graft is not retrieved from the insertion of the iliotibial band at the Gerdy's tubercle (Fig. 6.7). The idea is to keep its complete insertion on the tibia so that the isometric tension of the graft is preserved (Fig. 6.8).

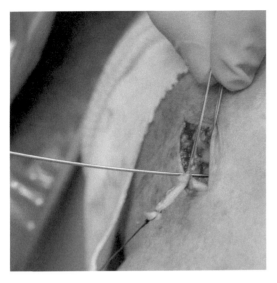

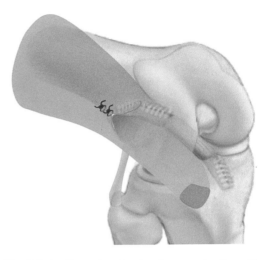

Fig. 6.7 An illustration showing the reconstruction with its attached part on the Gerdy's tubercle

Fig. 6.5 The relay wire is passed through the graft

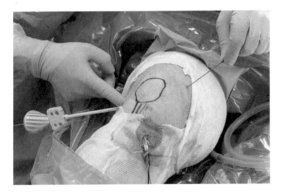

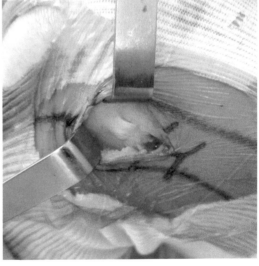

Fig. 6.6 The tension of the graft is checked while having the knee in extension position

Fig. 6.8 Final aspect

Take Home Messages

- The isometric point of the femoral fixation as well as positioning the knee at 20° and in neutral position are the two key points of this technique. Otherwise, the tensioning of the graft while pulling the tracking wire allows an optimal adjustment.

The Posterior Cruciate Ligament: PCL Reconstruction Using the Semitendinosus

7.1 Overview

For this rare type of surgery, we chose a technique close to that of the single four-strand semitendinosus graft for its easier reproducibility. The choice of a double bundle, closer to the anatomy, allows a better laxity control, in flexion as well as in extension. Here, risk taking must be minimal through the systematic usage of the image intensifier and passing the "killer turn" using a flexible graft.

7.2 The Single Four-Strand Semitendinosus Tendon Harvesting

Refer to the chapter on the single four-strand semitendinosus tendon harvesting technique.

7.3 Graft Preparation

The preparation is similar to that of the four-strand semitendinosus tendon harvesting technique but we use an additional endobutton to create a second femoral bundle.

Consequently, we obtain a Y-plasty (Fig. 7.1):

- one bundle and four strands at the tibia, and
- two bundles, one anterolateral and another posteromedial, with two strands each

The ideal total length is proximately 70 mm:

- 35–40 mm intra-articular.
- A minimal 15 mm in each tunnel.

Each bundle is measured: 6 mm on average for the AL and PM bundles and 9 mm on the tibia.

7.4 A Complete Tunnel Using the Image Intensifier

For us the posteromedial approach is optional. In fact, the killer-turn issue using the short hamstring graft is minor relatively to the use of the quadricipital or patellar tendons. It is then important to have an arthroscopic control of the retrospinal surface for the transplant passage. This direct vision however helps preparing the zone.

The cleaning of the retrospinal surface is done with the anteromedial port using 90° instruments: electric cautery probe, rugine, and a curette. In order to be sure that we have prepared the tibial tunnel emergence enough, especially distally, we can use the images of the image intensifier.

The point of the guide, inserted anteromedially, is placed on the retrospinal surface, 1.5 cm under the joint line, located with the laser mark (Fig. 7.2).

The guide is calibrated at 50–55° of inclination and impacted onto the medial surface of the tibia between the ATT and the insertion of the pes anserinus.

O. Courage et al., *Knee Arthroscopy*, https://doi.org/10.1007/978-3-030-82830-1_7

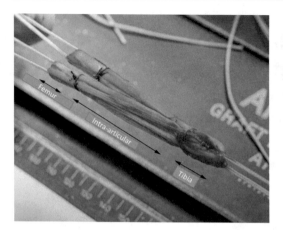

Fig. 7.1 A Y-plasty with two femoral bundles

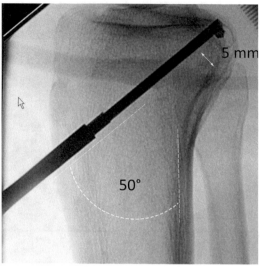

Fig. 7.3 Correct positioning control using the image intensifier

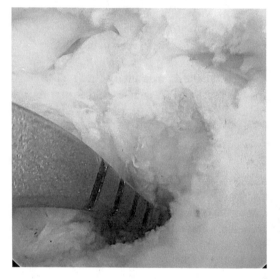

Fig. 7.2 Laser marking allowing for retrospinal gauging

A minimum distance of 5 mm should be reserved from the posterior wall to avoid its collapse while using the 9 mm auger (Fig. 7.3).

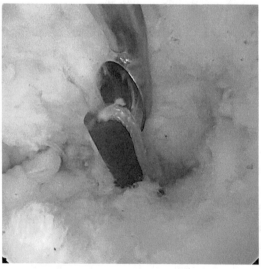

Fig. 7.4 Usage of the curette to pass the tracking wire anteriorly

Key Point: Tibial Tunnel Control Using the Image Intensifier

The guided pin is put under image intensifier control, directed slightly medially to laterally. An integrated spatula is inserted into the tibial guide to protect the posterior soft tissue.

The tunnel is then made using a 9 mm Flipcutter in a retrograde drilling and for a 35 mm length. This overlength allows the total entry of the graft in the tibial tunnel before we insert the bundles into the femur.

A relay wire is inserted into a stick and retrieved in an anterolateral "garage" portal with a curved curette that brings back the stick in the intercondylar fossa (Fig. 7.4).

7.5   Femoral Tunnels In-Out

Key Point: Tibial Tunnel Control with an Image Intensifier

The AL strand is at the roof of the fossa, at 11 o'clock for a left knee and 1 o'clock for a right knee. The footprint of the AL bundle is located at the most anterior and superior part of the PCL fibers insertion, at 2 mm interval from the medial cartilage (Figs. 7.5 and 7.6).

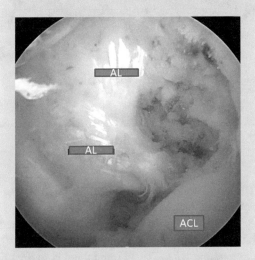

Fig. 7.5   Insertion of the two strands of the PCL

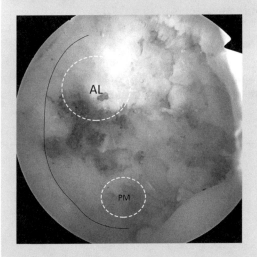

Fig. 7.6   After preparation of the fossa with a shaver

The femoral guide is calibrated at 90°, inserted via the anteromedial port, and positioned at each remnant of the PCL bundles to form its correspondent tunnel (Figs. 7.7, 7.8, 7.9, and 7.10).

Two tunnels are created with a 6 mm diameter and a length of 15 mm using a retrograde Flipcutter (Figs. 7.9, 7.10, and 7.11).

Note that we have to control the paratrochlear exit of the flipcutter arthroscopically to make sure not to damage the cartilage.

The three relay wires are retrieved with a shoulder grasping forceps from the same anterolateral port (Figs. 7.12 and 7.13).

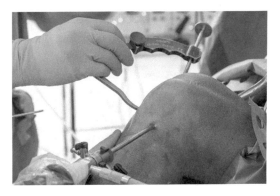

Fig. 7.7   Positioning of the outside-in guide through the anteromedial port

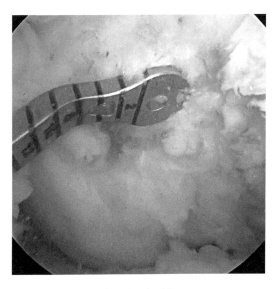

Fig. 7.8   Guide positioned at the AL remnant

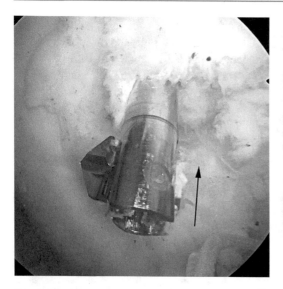

Fig. 7.9 Retrograde drilling with a Flipcutter

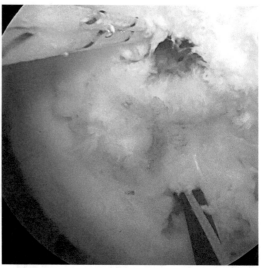

Fig. 7.11 Wire passage through the rigid stick

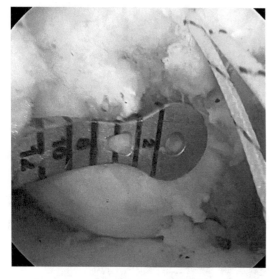

Fig. 7.10 Guide positioned on the PM remnant

7.6   Ascent, Tension Adjustment, and Transplant Fixation

The tibial endobutton is passed through its correspondent looped tracking wire.

The tibial part of the graft is first inserted intra-articularly then into the tibial tunnel using the tracking wire. The 35 mm tunnel is so important that it enables the entire graft to go in. This allows a better distinction between the two femoral strands (Figs. 7.14 and 7.15).

Then the AL and PM strands are inserted into their correspondent tunnels (Fig. 7.16).

One trick while passing the endobuttons through the tunnel is to hold the wires with a grasping forceps maintaining tension on these to

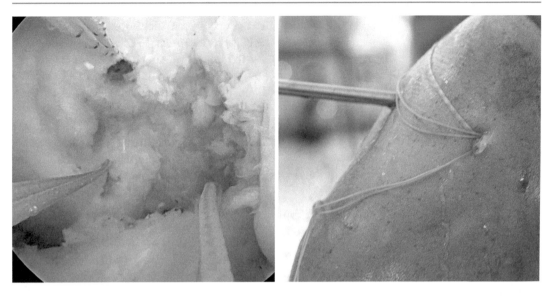

Figs. 7.12 and 7.13 Passage of the relay wires from the same anterolateral port

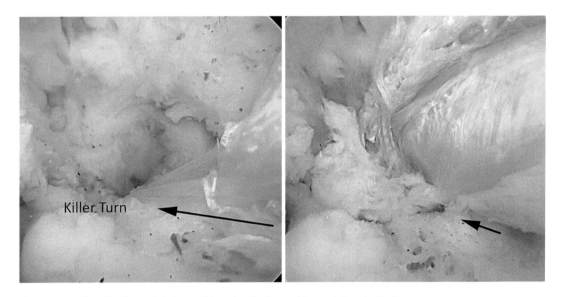

Figs. 7.14 and 7.15 The graft is inserted into the tibial tunnel beyond the wire limit

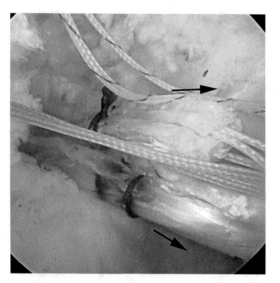

Fig. 7.16 The graft is entirely behind the tibia allowing a better visualization of the two strands

let the endobutton stick to the femoral bone to facilitate its ascension (Figs. 7.17, 7.18, and 7.19).

Like in the four-strand hamstring reconstruction, the tensioning is done progressively in order to make sure we have enough length of the graft in each tunnel.

The femoral strands are inserted 10 mm into the tunnels. The tibial part is then fixed and the strands tightened to the femur. Because of the length of the tibial tunnel, this order allows a reserve additional tension for the femoral tunnels (Figs. 7.20 and 7.21).

At the end of the intervention, we verify that the endobutton does not interfere with the femoropatellar joint (Figs. 7.22 and 7.23).

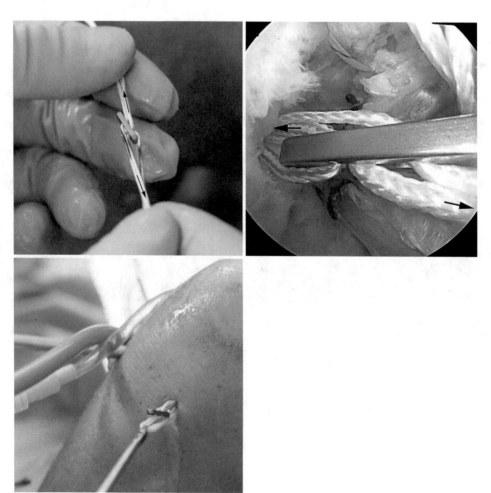

Figs. 7.17–7.19 Tensioning the wires from the two sides of the endobutton allows a better positioning and a better ascension

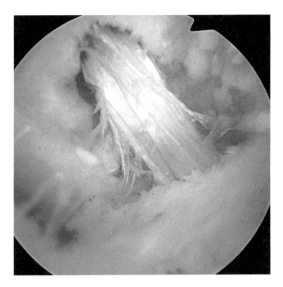

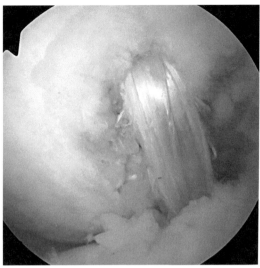

Fig. 7.20 The graft is inserted in each femoral tunnel until it reaches the 10 mm mark, then the tibial part is fixated

Fig. 7.21 Once the tibial strand is fixated, the femoral strands are then fixated. In this way, we are sure that we have enough graft tissue in both tunnels

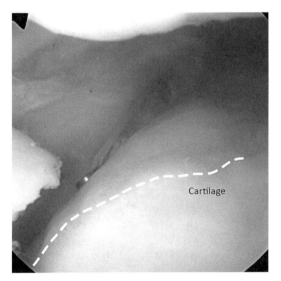

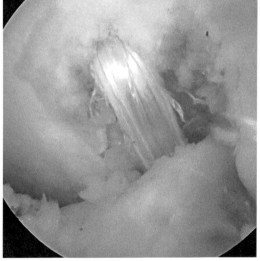

Fig. 7.22 Endobutton of the AL strand is kept within a distance from the cartilage

Fig. 7.23 Final aspect of the graft behind the native ACL

Take Home Messages

- The use of the image intensifier and the spatula protects the posterior soft tissue components.
- The complete entry of the graft into the tibial tunnel allows a better vision of the different femoral strands and an easier femoral ascent.

The MPFL: Double Bundle Reconstruction Using the Gracilis with Femoral and Tibial Rigid Fixations

8

8.1 Overview

Although the role of the medial patellar retinaculum and its avulsion are long well-known in patellar instability, the reconstruction of the medial patellofemoral ligament is but a new surgical technique that has been updated recently due to numerous anatomical studies. Henceforth, based on the same importance of the ATT osteotomy, this reconstruction is integrated into the arsenal of the primary intention surgery of patellar instability.

The MPFL is the primary passive restraint for the lateral patellar translation between 0° and 30° of flexion. It inserts onto the superior-medial aspect of the patella, anterior to the capsule. At the femur, it inserts posteriorly onto the medial femoral epicondyle just below the adductor tubercle.

The double bundle gracilis technique is derived from the one described by Schöttle thus enabling surgeons to reproduce the triangular aspect of the native medial patellar retinaculum with a broader insertion over the patella, while making a rigid fixation in the two extremities of the graft.

8.2 Patient Positioning

Patient positioning is classic with the knee at 90° of flexion (Fig. 8.1). The screen of the image intensifier is placed at the ipsilateral knee (Fig. 8.2).

We mark the location of the image intensifier with a tape after having the best lateral X-ray view possible. The draping is done taking into consideration covering the image intensifier and parking it closer to the head of the patient to have an easier access to the operating area where lie the pes anserinus, the medial border of the patella and the medial femoral condyle (Fig. 8.3).

8.3 Gracilis Tendon Harvesting and Length Verification

The harvesting of the gracilis can be done using the classic anterior approach or the posterior one.

We proceed with making several half hitch knots at the two extremities of the tendon for a 15 mm length.

Simulating the final position of the graft allows a better appreciation of its length (Fig. 8.3).

Allow a minimum of 18 cm in length for the transplant: 5 cm per bundle on average and at least 2 cm per tunnel.

8.4 Preoperative Skin Marking at the Fixation Sites

The incisions are 2 cm in length each at the patellar and femoral fixation sites (Fig. 8.4):

- At the superomedial border of the patella.
- Posteriorly to the medial epicondyle.

Fig. 8.1 Classic position of the patient with the knee at 90° of flexion and a lateral stress post

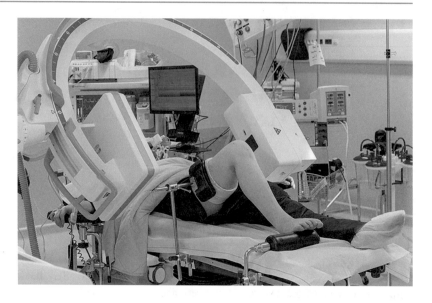

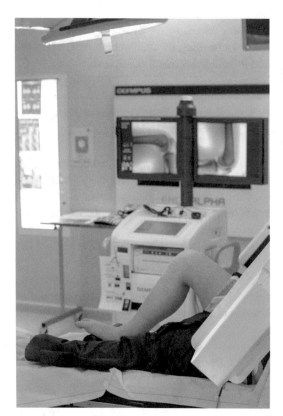

Fig. 8.2 Locating the best lateral X-ray view with an image intensifier and marking the location with a tape

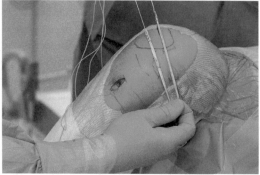

Fig. 8.3 Simulating the final position of the graft to be sure we have enough length

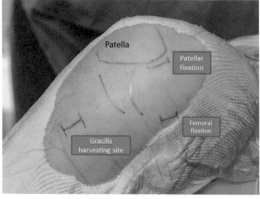

Fig. 8.4 Skin marking

8.5   Patellar Tunnel Fixation with Screws

The skin incision is small but should be sufficient to make sure that we are at the middle of the patellar thickness, in order to avoid a partial tunnel with an anterior or posterior wall collapse, which prevents a good fixation.

The palpation of the superior patellar border with hooked fingers helps visualize the patellar height (Fig. 8.5).

The good positioning can be confirmed with an X-ray.

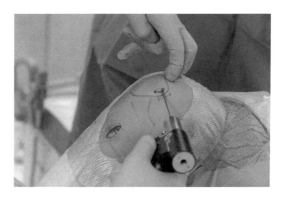

Fig. 8.5 Hooked fingers help visualize the patellar height and stabilize it while drilling

---

Key Point: The Patellar Fixation

The tunnels should be:

- At least 1 cm distant from one another to avoid tunnel collapse.
- Parallel and made with a 5 mm drill (Fig. 8.6).
- In the superior one-third of the patellar height.
- 20 mm in length.

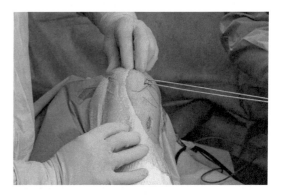

Fig. 8.6 The pins should be parallel

The fixation should be done with 24.75 cm diameter and 19.1 mm length screws used in shoulder surgery (Fig. 8.7).

We should check the good stability of these screws with a traction test on the grafts.

We should verify that the length of the transplant is sufficient and the Y aspect is reproduced (Fig. 8.8).

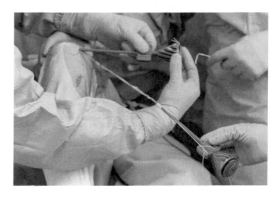

Fig. 8.7 Patellar fixation

Key Point: Positioning of the Femoral Tunnel

The difficulty in this operation lies in finding the isometric point of the ligament dictating the femoral tunnel position, allowing a maximal tensioning of the fibers at 30° of flexion.

8.6   Femoral Fixation with a Screw in a Complete Tunnel

Now is the most important part: the femoral part. The position of the tunnel is well described by Schöttle. The isometric point is located 5 mm distal from a tangent line to the posterior condyles and 5 mm anteriorly from a tangent line to the posterior diaphyseal femoral cortical wall (Fig. 8.9). This is done with the help of an image intensifier (Fig. 8.10). It is recommended that we do the skin incision with the help of the image intensifier because we have a tendency to do it too anteriorly.

The femoral tunnel is made using a 6 mm diameter cannulated drill into which we insert a trocar tip pin.

A nonabsorbable loop tracking wire is passed through the graft creating a double bundle aspect. It is then retrieved using a Kelly forceps from the femoral incision allowing the graft to pass into the intermediate space, between the articular capsule deeply and the fascia superficially.

The key here is to place the screw guided pin before the graft ascent in the tunnel to facilitate this process (Fig. 8.11). The guided pin is maintained in the tunnel throughout the time of the graft tensioning (Fig. 8.12).

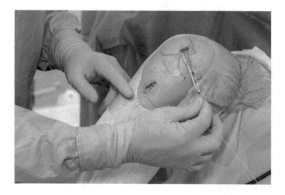

Fig. 8.8 Length verification with the two bundles

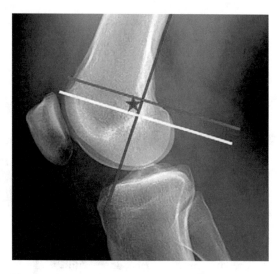

Fig. 8.9 Schöttle illustration allowing us to find the isometric point

Key Point: Graft Tensioning

The tensioning is done at 20° of flexion. While pulling the graft we should be able to feel the medialization of the patella but without excess. In fact, the patella should keep a transverse mobility to decrease the pressure on the medial facet, a source of postoperative pain. Thus, we should place the external facet in contact with the external border of the trochlea during fixation.

Fig. 8.10 Femoral positioning using the image intensifier

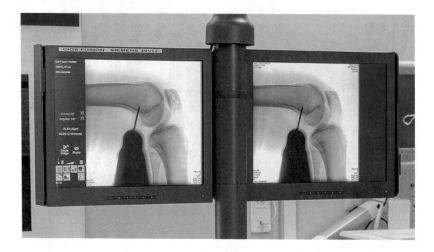

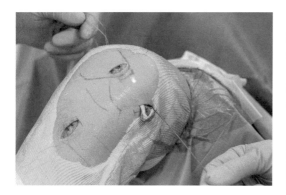

Fig. 8.11 The screw guided pin is inserted before the graft ascent in the tunnel to facilitate this process

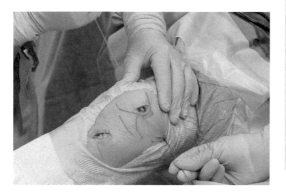

Fig. 8.12 The guided pin is left in place and the knee is flexed at 20°

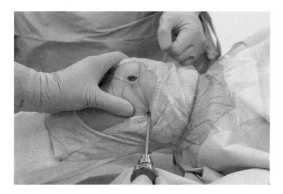

Fig. 8.13 Tensioning is maintained by the assistant and graft locking with the screw

The fixation is done with a 6 mm diameter and 23 mm length absorbable interference screw (Fig. 8.13).

Before closing, we should verify with our finger that the screw does not surpass the femoral cortical wall.

Take Home Messages

- Parallel drilling of the patellar tunnels.
- Control of the good stability of the graft in the patellar tunnels.
- Use the image intensifier to locate the isometric femoral point.
- Keep in mind not to have an excessive tension on the graft while fixating it, keep certain transverse mobility.
- Insert the guided pin before passing the graft in order to easily find the tunnel.
- Verify with the finger that the femoral screw does not pass the femoral cortical wall.

Annex A: Learning on the Simulator

As you have noticed all along this book, companionship is an extremely important element in the arthroscopic formation, but we should always keep abreast of the latest methods.

The learning curve could be considerably accelerated with the use of the arthroscopic simulators.

So we have acquired, more than 10 years ago, the arthroscopic simulator "VirtaMed."

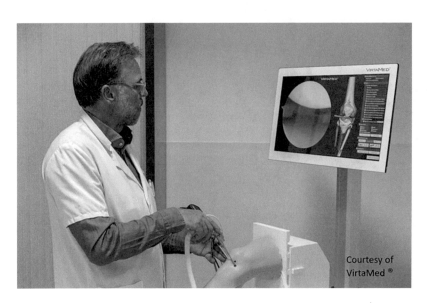

Courtesy of VirtaMed ®

Knee arthroscopy simulation. Courtesy of VirtaMed®

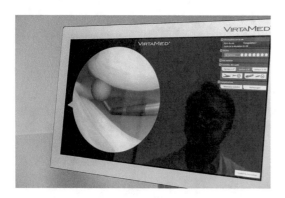

Exercising on triangulation using the VirtaMed

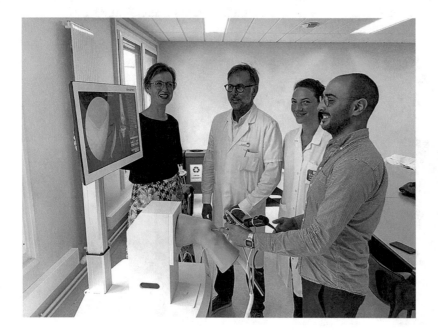

Team building and learning stimulation

This machine presents an arthroscopic reality highly sophisticated and the models offer a sensation so close to reality.

The basic exploration is acquired faster. The learning is gained progressively, by small successive steps in the operating room. For example, in the exploration mode, each compartment should be totally validated before passing to the next step.

By practicing to catch targets in a box or in the articulation, we acquire instinctively, like in video games, certain dexterity. That is why handling the instruments and their acknowledgment, like holding the scope or mastering the triangulation, is gained faster, in a few sessions only.

Simple interventions like in meniscectomies or more complex like ACL reconstruction are made too. These situations encountered help evaluate the duration needed in each operation and also learn from our mistakes: iatrogenic cartilage damage, unnecessary paths made by the scope and the instruments, bad positioning of the tunnels, etc.

The final report of each simulation mode shows us one's weaknesses in order to strengthen them.

Although this instrument is addressed to the young surgeons in formation, it can be compared to arthroscopic techniques once the dexterity is acquired. As a matter of fact, even for experienced surgeons, having to deal with this machine reveals some surprises, notably in terms of iatrogenic cartilage damaging induced in real-life surgery.

As perfect as it is, the simulation in arthroscopy is still at its beginnings. To which end will the catastrophe scenarios drawn by the simulator would reflect real-life confrontations in the operating room? In the future, these simulators will become essential for the continuous formation of the surgeon that is also present in the aviation or navigation world a long time ago, allowing each person to continue his improvement alongside his career.

Annex B: Graft Preparation During a Quadruple Stranded Semitendinosus Technique

Preparation on Operating Table

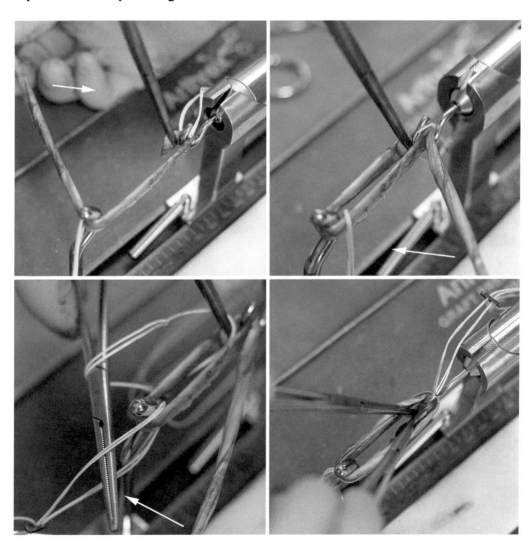

Figs. B.1–B.4 Passing the graft through the loops of the endobuttons using two Kocher forceps

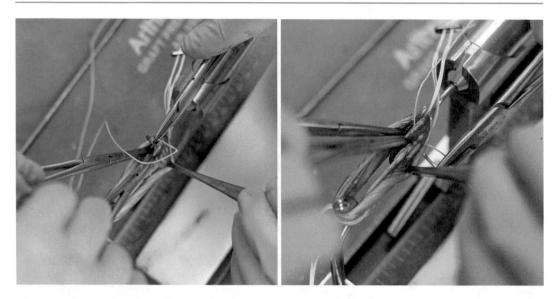

Figs. B.5 and B.6 FiberWire back and forth passage through one of the two bundles

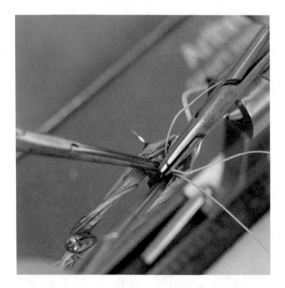

Fig. B.7 Simple passage without return in the other one

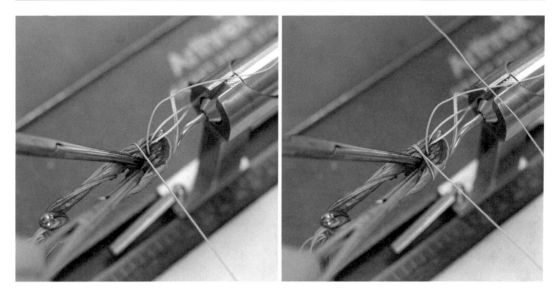

Figs. B.8 and B.9 Encircling twice the graft

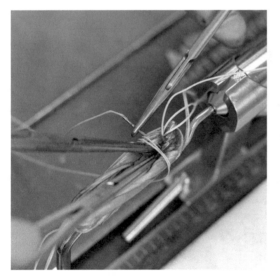

Fig. B.10 A return passage to exit in the middle of the graft

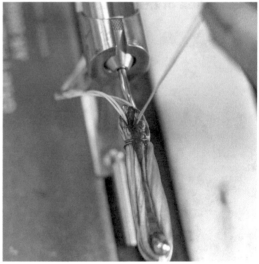

Fig. B.11 The two wires are tied between the two bundles

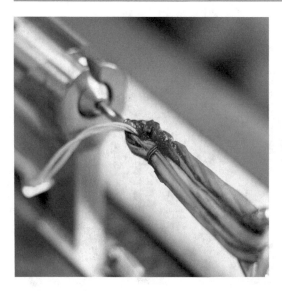

Fig. B.12 So the knot is hidden

Preparation of the Tibial Extremity

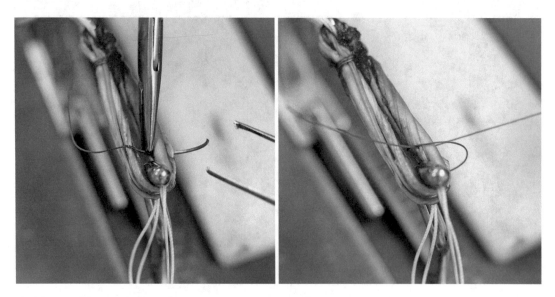

Figs. B.13 and B.14 Separated suturing of each bundle

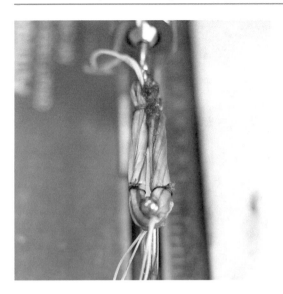

Fig. B.15 Final aspect of the graft

Printed in the United States
by Baker & Taylor Publisher Services